"If you want to cling to your excuses for not getting into and maintaining great overall physical condition, then don't buy Pat Flynn's *Strong ON!*. This book is a one-stop shop for your overall fitness plan (including diet), and it can be done in a manageable amount of time with minimal equipment. It sounds like it's on you to get in shape!"

—Jim Madden, PhD, professor of philosophy, former world Brazilian jiujitsu champion, and author of *Ageless Athlete*

"The Maestro of Minimalism does it again! Pat has put together the best dang collection of kettlebell workouts I've ever laid eyes on. This spectacular stash of routines is tough on weakness, gentle on the joints, and forges an uncompromising, jealousy-inducing physique that you'll be eager to show off any chance you get. If you get one book on kettlebell workouts this year, make it this one. Excuses off—*Strong ON!*"

—Aleks Salkin, author of *The No BS Kettlebell and Bodyweight Kickstart Program*

"Pat Flynn's book, *Strong ON!*, is, perhaps sadly, the book we all wanted in 2004. The clarity Pat shares of buying, using, learning, and coaching (. . . and sweating) fulfills our expectations of the magic promised by the kettlebell and the kettlebell community two decades ago. I'm asking out loud, 'Where was this book then?' Well, time only goes one direction, so here is the book now. Pat continues to amaze us with his sound (and simple) teaching points and the section on organizing training weeks is worthy of the university classroom. Of course, it's the workouts that most will look for . . . and Pat delivers here. I found this a fun read but overwhelmingly informative. If you have only room for one kettlebell book on your bookshelf, *Strong ON!* is the one you want."

—Dan John, author of *Never Let Go*

STRONG ON!

STRONG ON!

101 Minimalist Kettlebell Workouts
to Blast Fat, Build Muscle, and Boost
Flexibility—in 20 Minutes or Less

PAT FLYNN

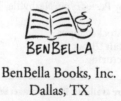

BenBella Books, Inc.
Dallas, TX

Strong ON! copyright © 2024 by Pat Flynn

BenBella Books, Inc.
10440 N. Central Expressway
Suite 800
Dallas, TX 75231
benbellabooks.com
Send feedback to feedback@benbellabooks.com

BenBella is a federally registered trademark.

Printed in the United States of America
10 9 8 7 6 5 4 3 2 1

Library of Congress Control Number: 2024025036
ISBN 9781637745410 (trade paperback)
ISBN 9781637745427 (electronic)

Editing by Claire Schulz and Scott Calamar
Copyediting by Jessica Easto
Proofreading by Rebecca Maines and Natalie Roth
Text design and composition by PerfecType, Nashville, TN
Cover design by Morgan Carr
Cover image © Shutterstock / Stocksnapper
Interior photography by Rebekah Ulmer
Printed by Lake Book Manufacturing

Special discounts for bulk sales are available. Please contact bulkorders@benbellabooks.com.

For my children

CONTENTS

INTRODUCTION

Growing up, like many kids in the '90s, my days were dominated by video games and the allure of tasty, unhealthy snacks. My main physical activities? Sitting and resting. As a result, I became noticeably heftier than my peers. It wasn't easy being the most rotund among my friends—or worse, rivals. It was, in fact, a source of repeated embarrassment. Quite often I found myself crafting imaginative excuses (like "Sorry, Mr. B, I need to . . . floss my cat") just to avoid gym class.

The turning point? Winning a wet T-shirt contest. As a dude.

See, during my middle and high school years, I was part of a rock band (you've likely never heard of us). My bandmates, who I naively considered friends, had a knack for playfully pointing out the keyboardist's and my most . . . robust features. One day, they held a mock election to decide who was the "Porker Supreme" between the two of us (how democratic, I know!). Being a typical middle schooler, I went along with this ridiculous scheme, albeit grudgingly. And thus, a memorable and painfully embarrassing story was memorialized in my little book of life.

Humiliating as this moment was, it did set a new trajectory for me, one with a far greater concern for health. So, this is not a sob story, ultimately; it's mostly just reporting.

Like pretty much everybody who sets out on some grand, life-changing fitness adventure, I was extremely confused about how and where to start—that is, how to lose weight and build muscle and then sustain it. My mother,

a devotee of the latest dieting fads, had an impressive collection of info-
mercial products and diet books amassed in the basement. I thought that
might be a good starting point. However, it quickly dawned on me that
the real challenge wasn't the scarcity of information but rather the overwhelming abundance of it—and much of it questionable. Everybody had
an opinion. Run or lift weights? Low fat or low carb? Multiple small meals
or extended fasting?

Ay yi yi.

See This?

Throughout this book, I've peppered in some boxes. These addi-
tions ultimately offer two reading paths: a straightforward one
for those wanting the core message and a detailed one for those
keen on understanding the principles shaping my advice, or just
making note about something I feel is helpful to share, even if
not essential.

But then a sort of fitness blessing was bestowed. While my buddy and
I drove around one day after school, we noticed a free trial lesson offered
at a local martial arts studio. We popped in, almost as a joke, because we
had nothing better to do. But the joke, as it happened, was quickly on me
because I loved every minute of it. I finally felt like I had found an outlet to
develop myself. So, I signed up. (Only problem was, I didn't have any money,
so I bartered cleaning bathrooms for tuition.)

Long story short, martial arts, specifically, tae kwon do, was when real
transformation started to happen. At least for me. I was lucky enough to
train under a real guru of sorts who steered me away from so many fitness
gimmicks and false starts and kept me focused on the proper fundamentals
of eating and effective lifting.

By the time I entered college, I could see my abs, a reality I never
thought possible just a few years earlier. I wasn't "huge," but I was fit. I had

dropped considerable weight, built a substantial amount of strength, and was well conditioned.

Immediately, I joined the collegiate tae kwon do team.

Somnath Sikdar, my coach at the time and now a good friend (best friend? We'll have to see what he gets me for Christmas), was an absolute specimen. He had all the physical features I wanted—ripped, explosive, densely muscled. He looked hard and hit harder. His secret? I *had* to find out.

At this time, my exercise routine was effective but cumbrous and somewhat wasteful. Som taught me about kettlebells and how I could reduce my exercise time substantially, which was important now that life was getting more hectic. Even when I was in college, I didn't have all the time in the world, and certainly I don't now. Efficiency was a selling point.

I'm not going to get into all the details of training with kettlebells now because, well, that's what this entire book is about. But I will say this: While I had a decent grasp of the fundamentals of effective exercise at this point, kettlebells allowed me to increase my efficiency magnificently and have, frankly, a lot more fun with the routines themselves. Training time decreased while results continued to increase, and I found myself becoming better conditioned overall for tae kwon do.

Here is my hope and aim for this book. I was fortunate to have all the fitness BS systematically eliminated by having a couple of good coaches—straight shooters with nothing purportedly magical to sell. I want to provide that same service for you. Coaches = shortcuts. Because a coach is like a trail guide: They can't walk the path for you, but they can chart the path and walk beside you, helping show the true way to real results, offering the necessary course corrections as various obstacles or impediments arise.

A NEVER-ENDING LIST OF FITNESS MYTHS

In the realm of fitness, there's a cacophony of claims, often touted with unwavering confidence, that are very likely, if not undeniably, untrue. These assertions, despite occasionally containing a nugget of truth or residing at the far end of extremities with reality located somewhere in between, lead to much confusion and many false starts.

For instance:

- "Eating [fat] [carbs] [frequently] [late at night] makes you fat."
- "Spot reduction works."
- "You need a gym membership to get fit."
- "Cardio is the holy grail of weight loss."
- "Crunches are the path to a flat stomach."
- "Lifting weights makes you bulky."
- "Breakfast is the most important meal of the day."
- "Breakfast is inconsequential."
- "You can offset a poor diet with exercise."
- "Soreness is the gauge of a productive workout."
- "Supplements are a surefire solution."
- "Supplements are perpetually futile."
- "You must exercise every single day."
- "You should steer clear of daily workouts."
- "Muscle magically transforms into fat when you cease exercising."
- "High-protein diets jeopardize your kidneys."
- "As you age, building muscle becomes an impossible feat."

And the list goes on.

What's the veritable truth amid this web of myths? Sometimes, it's a straightforward negation ("No, high-protein diets do not jeopardize your kidneys"). In other instances, the truth lies within the spectrum of two equally false or misleading assertions ("Some supplements, coupled with an effective exercise routine and balanced diet, can indeed provide benefits"). Occasionally, the matter is more nuanced ("While daily workouts are possible, prudent management of variables, particularly intensity, is key").

On the other hand, there are statements that, from a technical standpoint, are true but can be misleading or overly simplistic in practice. Take the claim that "all calories are created equal," for instance. It is accurate in the sense that a calorie is a unit of measure for energy. However, it's essential to recognize that not all calorie sources are equal in terms of their over-all impact on health and fitness. Foods rich in essential nutrients, fiber, and other advantageous compounds like antioxidants and fatty acids provide more comprehensive nutrition and better support overall health and fitness goals than calorie sources primarily composed of so-called empty calories—commonly found in the typical American diet. I mean, this is just common sense, right? Consider two individuals with equal calorie intake: One consumes a balanced diet of lean protein, fruits, vegetables, and healthy fats, while the other's diet consists solely of Keebler Fudge Shoppe cookies. Undoubtedly, their physical appearance, overall well-being, and quality of life will diverge significantly, despite sharing identical caloric intake.

IN SHORT, HERE'S WHAT TO EXPECT FROM THIS BOOK

Simple, no-nonsense instructions for minimalist fitness success. You won't just learn the basics here; you'll discover how to piece together workouts into an effective weekly plan based on your goals. Moreover, I've included 101 straightforward, written-out kettlebell workouts, which you can just plug and play. Why 101? I don't know. I just like uneven numbers. They smell nice.

In addition, I offer a unique and somewhat internet famous 300 Swings Kettlebell Challenge for you to indulge whenever you feel daring. Also, I share the simplest yet oh-so-scientific approach to eating that I know how to give.

Finally, I should probably say something (more) about myself. It's important, I feel, to make known that I am not just another guy with pretty genetics (my genetics suck, lol) offering trendy fitness advice online. Instead, I am somebody who had their life truly transformed by coaches who had—out of respect for themselves and others—zero time for BS, and I became ferociously inspired to pay it forward.

As you'll learn in the next chapter, my philosophy about fitness—the philosophy of *Strong ON!*—is both minimalist (getting the most from the least) and generalist (being good to great at almost everything). I'll explain each in detail, but I can already hear the skepticism about the latter point: "Are you suggesting it's better to be a jack-of-all-trades than a master of one?" Not exactly. A generalist can master multiple domains without being the absolute best in any single one. Mastery and being the "world's best" aren't synonymous; the generalist—or expert-generalist—thrives in this space: jack-of-many-trades and master of . . . quite a few!

Case in point: me. I'm a proud generalist. In fact, I penned the book on generalism, *How to Be Better at (Almost) Everything* (BenBella, 2019) and have authored works spanning from fitness to philosophy.* My life mirrors my eclectic writing: from a master of science in philosophy to a black belt in tae kwon do, from a music creator—I cover '80s party metal solos on You-Tube (hit the QR code below for my cover of Van Halen's "Eruption") and gig heavily with my Milwaukee-area band Poundcake—to an entrepreneur who has run an online business for nearly two decades, allowing me and my wife to homeschool our five children. Life is busy. But good and full.

In the realm of fitness, I consistently keep my body fat below 10 percent without resorting to medical intervention or "special vitamins." My capabilities—if we can call them that—include executing muscle-ups, pistol squats, and one-arm push-ups. Besides, I boast commendable stats in classic lifts—a testament being my recent triumph in a pull-up competition at a local smoothie shop where I achieved twenty-nine (strict!) reps, a little reminder to myself that "Dad's still got it." While I don't chase accolades at national fitness events, put me in a decathlon of fitness challenges—strength, mobility, and endurance—and there's a good chance I'll rank at the top, even when up against hyperspecialists. They'll definitely get me at some things, but probably I'll get them at most things.

---

* As of writing this book, my most recent works in philosophy include the popular level book *The Best Argument for God* (Sophia, 2023) and the scholarly article "Is Grounding Essentially Ordered Causation?" (the *Review of Metaphysics*). My other fitness-related works include *Paleo Workouts for Dummies*, *Fast Diets for Dummies*, and *Paleo All-in-One for Dummies*—all pretty good books, I think, just with admittedly terrible titles.

So, in short, I do *a lot* of stuff, and I do all of it—if I may say so—well. People hire me to teach them things, from fitness to business to writing to music, because they see I have command of the material. I am not, nor have I ever claimed to be, the best in the world at any one thing that I do; I'm not the best at fitness (whatever that means), the best writer, the best musician, or the best martial artist. I strive for greatness, not best-ness, and you should, too. Why? Because it's easier and better and almost certainly healthier to be electively diverse than it is to be the best in the world at any one thing.

Important clarification: I'm not proclaiming unparalleled excellence but rather highlighting achievable broad-spectrum success, which is not reserved just for prodigies. *I'm* just a regular guy—really! (If you recall, I failed on the advice of picking rich, genetically gifted parents and not getting fat in the first place.) I didn't have enormous early fitness advantages, but I did eventually get some awesome coaches who provided practical advice and encouragement—and that is just what I hope to provide for you. Because the cliché, at least in my case, is true: If I can do it, then anybody can do it, at any time. Including you.

Let's begin.

1

ALL FITNESS IN A
SINGLE SENTENCE

To thrive in fitness, do this: *Lift with gusto several times a week, nearing technical failure to boost strength and muscle; make metabolic resistance training your time-saver; walk and stretch daily; feast on natural foods and protein, keeping a tab on calories; go easy on booze; and get some quality shut-eye.*

In that admittedly complex sentence lies the road map to fitness. Adhere to these guidelines and witness transformative results. Stray from them, and you're in uncertain territory. (To be clear, these are broad principles, compatible with a wide range of specific exercise and diet strategies.)

The aim of this chapter is clarity. As I mentioned in the introduction, the fitness journey can be obscured by overwhelming (mis)information. I'll delineate the foundational principles affirmed by science and personal experience.

Let's start here: There is a saying in fitness circles that there is no one-size-fits-all approach. While the sentiment is something I appreciate—insofar as we're trying to invite everyone to success and suggesting there is room for personal preference—it's not entirely accurate. We really *do* know

what works for people—all people, always, and in all places—and some of
these things are immutable truth, like training against resistance if you
want to grow muscle and controlling calories if you want to drop fat. In that
sense, what works is just what works, and nobody is exempted. However,
one can adhere to universal principles through a variety of programs, and
that's where there is considerable room for personal preference and lifestyle
considerations. Yes, you need to resistance train if you want to build muscle,
but you can resistance train with kettlebells, barbells, dumbbells, or your
own body weight. Moreover, you can resistance train through different set
and rep schemes and experience similarly awesome results. So long as the
basic principles are implemented, and consistently so, success can be found
through a surprisingly large number of different approaches (kettlebell or
dumbbell, barbell or body weight, heavy weight and lower rep, lower weight
and higher rep, etc.). However, if the basic principles are not implemented,
and consistently so, no approach will fare better than any other.

Same with diet: So long as certain targets (e.g., caloric) are hit, it doesn't
matter so much what specific approach you take—Mediterranean, intermittent fasting, Paleo, keto, vegetarian, etc.—again, so long as the principles are
implemented, and consistently so.

AN IMMEDIATE CLARIFICATION

Unfortunately, brevity can sometimes cloud clarity. While I champion
natural foods, I don't categorically condemn all processed ones. In fact,
some processed items, like certain protein supplements (we'll discuss
these later), are undeniably beneficial despite being "processed." The real
emphasis here is on favoring foods close to their natural form—like lean
meats, fruits, veggies, nuts, and seeds—while being wary of items with
extensive ingredient lists that lack substantial nutritional value while being
extremely easy to overconsume. (I'm casting a side-eye at you, Mr. Sour
Cream and Onion Potato Chip. With ridges? Get out of here!)

I understand there is nothing particularly sexy or, for many, revolutionary about these statements. But we have to be absolutely clear about why people—including people consistent in their efforts—do not get the results they want in and out of the gym. It comes down to this: Even if they are consistent, they simply don't work hard enough. They train without sufficient intensity or focus—they put in the reps, but the reps are not effective reps.

There is another saying often heard in fitness circles that the best program is the one you can stick with. But again, consistency is only (to use philosopher speak) a necessary but not sufficient condition for success. One can, as many do, apply consistent efforts to a mediocre training plan and wind up pretty much in the same place a year, five years, ten years from now as they are today. We all know people like this. They show up and they *do* put in the work, consistently so, but it is not the sort of work that makes much difference. Please don't get me wrong. All activity is good for *health*—on that front, almost no physical activity is ineffective in the sense of being wasteful, though certainly one can be more or less efficient, as with anything. Here I am talking about wanting to get stronger, build muscle, and lean out. You need to be consistent, yes, but you also need to be accurate (choose the right exercises) and intense (work hard at them).

So, the best program isn't just the one you stick with *but the one you push yourself hardest in*, ensuring exercises are both challenging and beneficial. That last part matters quite a bit, since just because an exercise is "difficult" doesn't mean it's beneficial. Many exercises are difficult yet amazingly useless—as in not easy to perform but mostly, if not entirely, a waste of time for getting the results most people want. Performing a single-leg dumbbell row upon a BOSU ball* is, for many people, rather difficult. But is this exercise really the best use of one's time if they're trying to maximize strength and muscle gain? Definitely not. The point isn't that there is not, nor could never be, a justifiable purpose for exercises like the one named above. It's just that many people perform them simply because they feel (or look)

---

* If you don't know what any of that is, that may, quite honestly, be for the best.

difficult when sticking with the basics (squats, deadlifts, presses) would be far more effective. Remember, foundational exercises are foundational for a reason.

Again, my plan is to make all this simple for you. In the coming chapters, I will begin to spell out fundamental kettlebell exercises and describe how to perform them optimally. You won't have to guess when it comes to exercise selection—I'll do all of that for you when it comes to the workout programming. Nevertheless, I feel it's important for you to understand what's guiding my hand on this and why I am not a "variety for variety's sake" kind of guy. Generally, fewer exercises done with greater intensity are better for everyone, especially when those exercises are the big compound lifts we know get the best overall results.

Clear so far? I hope this brief articulation of Immutable Fitness Truth is at once grounding and liberating. Grounding in that it makes clear what *generally* must be done if serious, sustainable progress is to be made, liberating in that it does not restrain you to a single *specific* approach.

In summary, people often fail on a program not because the program didn't work but because they didn't work the program. They didn't understand the underlying principles and, hence, failed to implement them. It's often as simple as they just didn't push hard enough in the exercises they were doing, not that the sets or reps they were doing were the wrong number or anything like that. Because here's the truth: You can build strength and muscle with sets using very low reps (five) or rather high reps (twenty), but what matters is that you push right up to failure for whatever rep range you're using—if strength and muscle are what you want. If you don't consistently apply the principle of sufficient intensity (working close to failure), then any approach you take will likely fail, or at least not efficiently progress you, whereas if you do appreciate and consistently implement the principle of sufficient intensity, then almost any lifting approach you take can succeed.

So yes, principles. Principles are the thing. And in the simplest possible terms, the principles are:

- **For strength and muscle:** Lift weights with intensity and eat protein while increasing calories.
- **For conditioning and fat loss:** Lift weights with intensity and eat protein while decreasing calories.

EFFECTIVE REPS, QUALIFIED

Let's add a touch of nuance to the idea that muscle building can be achieved across a wide range of rep counts. While it's true that you can technically build muscle with various rep schemes, it's important to consider practicality—obviously.

When you opt for higher rep sets, approaching twenty or more reps, it's worth noting that you'll need to perform a considerable number of repetitions before reaching the "effective reps" range, where you approach muscle failure. Is it doable? Absolutely. But if you're aiming for time-efficient training, it may not be the most practical approach.

In the spirit of minimalist training, I often find the sweet spot for muscle building lies within the eight- to fifteen-rep range. This range strikes a balance between the number of reps needed to reach the effective zone and time efficiency. It's not a hard and fast rule, but it can help streamline your muscle-building efforts.

THE SCIENCE OF IT ALL

Numerous studies indicate that effective results can be achieved with minimal time in the gym, given the right intensity and focus. For instance, one meta-analysis examined the effects of single-set versus multiple-set training. It concluded that for short-term interventions (a fancy way of saying that people are put on a program of some sort), the outcomes of both methods are the same. However, for longer-term interventions and advanced subjects aiming to optimize strength gain, multiple-set strategies are superior. For example:

- **Strength:** A single heavy set, one to four times per week, can considerably improve strength.[1]
- **Health:** Thirty to sixty minutes of lifting weekly can have significant health benefits.[2]
- **Muscle:** While ten sets per muscle group per week is often recommended, even five to nine sets can yield around 80 percent of the same results.[3]

In other words, "science" says you don't have to hit the ideal to hit something absolutely worthwhile and save yourself considerable time.

The takeaway from all this? Push yourself. Because if you're going to train less, you must work harder. Minimalist training demands maximal effort. Remember: no junk sets.

While this book presents a unique fitness approach, it's not the sole method to attain strength, leanness, health, and resilience. Rather, it is crucial to understand the foundational principles to ensure proper application. That said, I've witnessed countless individuals thrive using the Strong ON! approach—that is, the approach of striving for a generalist (good to great at many things) outcome via a minimalist (effective and efficient) methodology. It's adaptable to various lifestyles, encompasses all foundational fitness elements, and offers both challenge and enjoyment. Notably, it's time savvy, with main workouts concluding in roughly twenty minutes. Our unique approach emphasizes kettlebells, though it's not limited to them.

Weightlifting for . . . Weight Loss?

Real quick, let me address a point that might sound immediately counterintuitive to many people, which is the idea of using weightlifting to lose weight. After all, isn't weightlifting all about gaining mass? Well, it can be. However, weightlifting offers far more than just muscle growth and strength gains. At its core, weightlifting transforms your body into a more metabolically active machine. Here's why: Muscle and strength are "expensive"—they consume energy. This means weightlifting helps you burn more calories automatically (while lounging about), rather than just manually (while exercising).

Simply put, the more muscle you have, the more energy you use. Just like a car, the bigger the engine (or muscles), the more fuel (or calories) it burns, even when idling (or doing daily activities).* For vehicles, a bigger engine is seen as less efficient, but when it comes to burning calories, this is the kind of inefficiency we desire. Weightlifting is the key to achieving it.

So, against popular belief, prolonged, slow-paced cardio isn't the gold standard for body transformation or fat loss. Don't get me wrong: A leisurely morning walk is super beneficial for overall health and definitely complements fat-burning routines. All I'm saying is it's not the most effective strategy when juxtaposed with rigorous resistance training.

Here's a critical point: Your exercise regimen to either gain or lose weight can, and often should, look quite similar. *It's not so much exercise or activity selection as it is the calorie intake that determines whether you gain or lose body mass.* For example, when you lift intensely and consume more calories, you're likely to gain muscle (and to some inevitable extent, fat). On the flip side, with the same intense lifting but fewer calories, you shed fat (and to some inevitable extent, muscle). This isn't to say that the two exercise phases are, or must be, identical, but they definitely can and almost certainly should share a foundational approach. For example, while focusing on fat loss, it may be beneficial to include more cardio, like walking or other endurance routines; when targeting muscle gains, you may want to perform more overall lifting volume. Nevertheless, these are largely nuanced adjustments to fine-tune your strategy, but otherwise the general approach is the same whether you want to gain or lose weight: Lift weights, eat protein, and adjust calories as needed.

Another prevalent misconception about weightlifting is the fear of becoming overly bulky, reminiscent of NFL linebackers or the Hulk or

---

* I borrow this analogy from coach Nick Tumminello. For more on the science of strength training and its benefits for fat loss, see his book *Strength Training for Fat Loss*.

something like that. This notion is largely a myth. Even individuals who purposely aim to bulk up find it to be a rather challenging, prolonged process. Achieving a massive bodybuilder-like physique just by lifting weights is a serious misconception. It demands a huge amount of dedication, a highly tailored training routine (different from what we're prescribing here), generous calorie consumption, and to be sure, a certain genetic predisposition. For the majority, weightlifting—paired with balanced nutrition—delivers just what most people want, most of the time: a leaner physique, chiseled muscles, and functional (as in, actually useful!) strength.

THE STRONG ON! PHILOSOPHY: GENERALIST AND MINIMALIST

We've just spent time talking about fitness (and some dietary) fundamentals. Let me now focus on my specific approach to getting these fundamentals in place and the controlling principles, if you will, that guide the decisions I make when putting together the specific plans, workouts, and recommendations in this book.

My philosophy when it comes to fitness—that is, the philosophy of Strong ON!—is this: Become an expert-generalist by being a fitness minimalist. Let me explain each of these in turn.

What Generalism Is

Generalism, in essence, is being good to great (or at least fairly competent) at whole bunches of stuff. Physically, it means being capable of, and ready for, whatever life throws at you, and maybe being the best guy or gal in your neighborhood (though maybe only in your neighborhood) at pull-ups and squats. The fitness generalist isn't fixated on hyperspecialization; they don't pine to clinch world titles in powerlifting or bodybuilding competitions. Instead, they aspire for a balanced prowess: lean but muscled, functionally strong, agile, limber, pain-free, and energetic. What's more, the generalist wants health and fitness to be mutually harmonious.

That's important because fitness isn't health. Fitness is the ability to complete a task whereas health is something like the ideal interplay between organs and bodily systems. People can get good at completing tasks while expensing health. Just think of professional powerlifters and bodybuilders, many of whom wind up on the operating table because of their efforts, suffering half a lifetime of serious injuries and illnesses or worse. Yet, nobody would deny they are fit, in the sense of being able to lift an extreme amount of weight, but their fitness pursuits actually caused them to be unhealthy.

The generalist is against this. Minimally, fitness should never detract from health. Preferably, fitness should enhance one's health. For many people, that's the number one thing they want from a fitness program, anyway (that and looking leaner and more muscled). No doubt, many people want to look a certain way, but they also want to feel a certain way. They want to feel healthy, and hopefully that is because they *are* healthy.

So, the generalist makes sure that fitness and health are never at odds—that we increase our ability to complete tasks only to the extent that we become more vibrant and resilient overall. Usually, it's when people hyperspecialize that health starts getting written off for fitness. Not with us.

How to Be Better at (Almost) Everything

While this book focuses on becoming a fitness generalist, if you're interested in developing and stacking skills in a range of disciplines, be sure to subscribe to my YouTube channel @HowtoBeBetteratEverything and get the book at HowtoBeBetterBook.com.

What Minimalism Is

Okay, so if generalism is the outcome, then minimalism is the method.

The minimalist, really, is just anyone who wants to maximize results with minimum input. Said another way, the minimalist is someone constantly striving to hit the ideal intersection between effectiveness (doing the right things) and efficiency (doing things right). Obvious, right? I mean, who would ever want to work ineffectively or inefficiently? Still, the point is not about what we want but what we are able to get. I'm assuming you want minimalism with fitness—that we are agreed upon. My job is to show you how to get it. That's the entire point of this book: fitness—real fitness, without gimmicks or fads—done fast.

EFFECTIVENESS VERSUS EFFICIENCY

To illustrate the difference between effectiveness and efficiency, consider this rather mundane example. Suppose you want to build upper-body strength and decide—for whatever reason—to follow a running program. Well, you may have a very well-designed running program, and you may also have an extremely slick and efficient running technique. Nevertheless, running is just not an effective effort for building upper-body strength—obviously. So, efficiency may be at play with effectiveness missing; you might be doing something quite well without that something making sense for the goal you want to achieve. On the other hand, suppose you decide to perform military presses to build upper-body strength, but your technique is quite poor and you are failing to perform enough reps or use a sufficient amount of weight. In this case, we have something that is effective and does make sense for the goal, but it's being performed poorly and inefficiently, ultimately slowing or stalling progress. All to say: The true minimalist is constantly seeking to maximize effectiveness, by picking the best efforts for the job, and efficiencies, by performing those efforts well.

Let's return to that point for a minute. Taking the minimalist approach means trying to make your efforts economical, but of course what counts as economical depends on the outcome you desire to achieve. In which case, minimalism doesn't (necessarily) mean doing *very little*; minimalism means doing *the least*. Sometimes the least is a lot, if the goal is, say, a big one. The minimalist just doesn't want to be wasteful, so they apply the minimum effective dose—time, energy, money, etc.—to get the effect they want and not a smidge more.

In other words, minimalism is not the object of our fitness efforts. Minimalism is the means. The object is generalism.

Figuring out what the minimum effective dose *is* might not always be possible until you've spent a lot of time practicing something, learning what works and what doesn't. That's why coaches are important—hopefully, they have already figured that stuff out for you, and they can guide you on being as effective and efficient as possible. I've done that for you, for fitness, anyway. Aren't I swell?

I could belabor these points, but that would be, I think, inconsistent with my minimalist promise. So let me just sum up and then we can press on. This book is about forging expert-generalists with respect to fitness—people who are leaner, stronger, and harder to kill—through the minimum effective dose of exercise. I want you to be good to great at lots of stuff, physically speaking, and I want to save you tons of time, ensuring no effort is anything less than a significant advance toward making you the person you want to be.

LOWERING BARRIERS TO ENTRY

In one sense, this book is extremely slim, easy reading. I get to the point quickly—"Do this, and here's why"—so *you* can get to acting on it. In another sense, this book is rather meaty, since it includes a substantial number of workouts. Fortunately, this hefty collection of kettlebell routines is either plug and play or grab and go (depending on which plan you choose), so it will not demand hours of additional reading—it will save you the time you'd otherwise spend thinking through and designing things for yourself. Again, all in the service of minimalism, removing barriers to entry, and success.

KETTLEBELLS 101

My first encounter with kettlebells was through Som (remember Som, from the introduction?), my tae kwon do coach. At the time, I was immersed in traditional lifting using barbells and dumbbells, which served me well. Nevertheless, my coach recognized an opportunity for me to optimize my training and suggested I integrate kettlebells into my regimen.

It was love at first lift.

My first kettlebell session involved a few basic exercises we'll explore later. This experience made it evident (to me, anyway) that kettlebells could significantly enhance my training efficiency, catering to both my hectic schedule and my pursuit of functional intensity. The kettlebell, I immediately realized, was just the right tool for the fitness minimalist.

WHY THE KETTLEBELL IS THE MINIMALIST'S ULTIMATE SECRET TRAINING WEAPON

Kettlebells' suitability for training complexes, combos, and chains is particularly striking. Picture this: seamlessly transitioning between exercises with minimal rest, allowing for a comprehensive workout training various muscle groups and energy systems in a succinct time frame. This epitomizes the essence of kettlebells—maximizing outcomes with minimal resources.

While it's certainly possible to use other equipment or body weight for similar complex workouts, the distinct design and inherent characteristics of the kettlebell differentiate it. This "cannonball with a handle" is seriously so well suited for both explosive movements, such as swings and snatches, and intense grind exercises, like presses and squats. Achieving the desired intensity using only body weight can be challenging, and while other equipment like barbells can easily reach high intensity, they lack the kettlebell's versatility because of their cumbersome nature.

In essence, consider the kettlebell the Swiss Army knife of functional fitness. While the kettlebell may not outperform every type of equipment in every aspect—barbells remain unparalleled for achieving peak deadlift strength—it's adept in various domains and especially useful for metabolic resistance training (more on that in a moment).

In fitness, as in life, it's about leveraging the right tool for the task at hand. Surely, with perseverance, one could dig a sizable hole using a spoon, but wouldn't a shovel be more appropriate?

In today's fitness realm, hyperbolic marketing claims are rampant. As for me, I aim for transparency and authenticity with my audience. Here's the candid truth: While kettlebells aren't the only route to fitness success, they're undeniably efficient, effective, and enjoyable based on my personal experience. Fortunately, you're a levelheaded person, not prone to marketing hype—I can see that. So, I suspect what I've said is all you need to get excited about training with kettlebells.

A PERHAPS UNNECESSARY DISCLAIMER

Everyone should be concerned about conflicts of interest when it comes to people promoting fitness ideas—there's a lot of shady stuff out there. Mine, fortunately, are notably few. First, while I do run a business selling

fitness information—largely programs and coaching that frequently feature kettlebell workouts—I do not sell kettlebells themselves, nor am I
sponsored or endorsed by any kettlebell brand, at least not at the time of
writing this book. Even if I were, I believe in prioritizing well-evidenced
fitness approaches over trendy or profitable ones. In simple terms, I offer
kettlebell-based programs and challenges because I genuinely believe in
their effectiveness, use them myself, and have seen excellent results with
my clients.

YOUR KETTLEBELL TOOLKIT—COMMON Q & A'S ON EQUIPMENT, EXERCISES, AND REST

Okay, before proceeding, let me go on cleanup duty by quickly hitting several questions commonly asked about kettlebell training. If you've never
picked up a kettlebell before, I suspect you will find this section helpful since
I will be assuming zero prior experience.

How many kettlebells should I get? To get started with this book, I
recommend getting at least three kettlebells—something light, something
medium, and something heavy. If you can swing it (pun!), you could even
double up on each of those bells, which will make the double kettlebell
workouts immediately accessible.

Of course, light, medium, and heavy are ambiguous specs, so let me
clarify. I want you to have a kettlebell that can challenge you (see the next
question to get an idea of what I mean by "challenge") for lower rep sets
(two to five reps) on exercises like squats and presses; I want you to have a
kettlebell that can challenge you for higher rep sets (six to twelve reps) on
exercises like squats and presses; and I want you to have a kettlebell that
you can use to perform multiple reps of exercises like swings for extended
periods—for example, fifteen to thirty seconds.

Obviously, no general recommendation is going to be a perfect fit for
everyone, but from experience, I can tell you the following sets are quite
effective as starter packs for beginners:

For women: 8 kg, 12 kg, 16 kg

For men: 12 kg, 16 kg, 24 kg

In the workouts in this book, you'll find the weight recommendations for women often range from 8 to 16 kg; for men, from 12 to 24 kg. Again, adjust upward or downward as you desire, whatever makes sense for your body structure (if you're naturally bigger or smaller) or feel your experience and general background fitness levels allow (and by the dictates of common sense). For example, if you're new to kettlebells but have a fair bit of time under your belt spent resistance training, you may want to begin with a slightly heavier set. Ultimately, as you run the workouts and get a better feel of the various exercise techniques, you'll develop a better idea of exactly what weights to get to appropriately challenge yourself. Don't stress about this—things always fit better over time, and starting out, it's okay to begin with an approximation.

How much weight should I use? Often, I'll provide you with an exercise in the workout to base your weight selection on. For example, you might see me suggest using "a weight that is between your 2- and 5-rep pressing max." This means you should choose a weight that allows you to complete between two to five reps before reaching technical failure. I offer ranges to provide flexibility in weight selection, considering that kettlebells may not always come in small increments (they often increase in 4 kg increments). Sometimes, you'll need to get as close as possible to the recommended weight without it being a perfect match. That's fine, as long as you're not significantly off the mark. Here's a general rule of thumb: When it comes to strength and muscle work, it's better to lean toward heavier weights (even if it occasionally results in missing a rep or two, but no more than that!). On the other hand, when it comes to conditioning work, it's okay to opt for weights on the lighter end of the recommended range to ensure you can complete all reps effectively.

How much rest should I take? This might be getting a little ahead of ourselves, since we haven't yet gotten to either the programming or the workouts, but it's a common question, so let me just address it now. Unless otherwise specified, rest between rounds of complexes should always be "as little as you need, but as much as you need to feel strong and confident going into your next set." Again, for strength and muscle work, better to lean toward a little more rest insofar as it allows you to work harder than you otherwise would with each set (i.e., lifting more weight or hitting all the reps). However, for conditioning work, you might want to compress the rest more to increase the relevant challenge. If you're someone who needs a "hard" recommendation, then keep most rest periods between one and three minutes. Note, however, that some workouts, like "every minute on the minute" (EMOM) routines, have fixed rest intervals—those will be obvious when you see them.

What are the best kettlebell exercises for beginners? Really and truly, the exercises taught and prescribed in this book are best. That said, they aren't just for beginners. Mastery, after all, is arguably about moving deeper into the basics, not further away from them. I generally perform the same fundamental kettlebell exercises today as I did starting out, all those many years ago.

Can kettlebells help with building muscle? Yes, absolutely. See the program in this book on exactly that.

Is kettlebell training suitable for all ages? Yes, it definitely is. Assuming one is cleared for regular exercise and attentive to proper (consistent) technique, people of all ages can benefit from kettlebell training by experiencing enhanced strength, lean muscle tissue, endurance, and mobility.

What Is Failure?

Technical failure is the point where you start noticing a significant decrease in rep quality, such as a drop in speed, or when you begin making compensatory movements to complete the reps. Absolute failure is when the weight becomes immovable for your body, regardless of any compensation or alteration of technique.

METABOLIC RESISTANCE TRAINING

Metabolic resistance training (MRT) has been gaining traction in the fitness world—and for a good reason. MRT is a potent training approach that simultaneously bolsters strength, enhances lean muscle development, maximizes calorie burn, and boosts overall work capacity (that is, the ability to perform and sustain physical activity). At its essence, MRT involves engaging in a series of compound movements, often back-to-back with minimal breaks. These can be done using heavy weights or by moving lighter weights more rapidly—two primary avenues to increase strength.

The multifaceted benefits of MRT are worth noting. Such sessions often target multiple muscle groups, while enhancing both aerobic capacities (like the sustained, talk-through activities such as walking) and anaerobic capabilities (intense, breath-stealing exercises like sprinting). Moreover, by extending the duration of resistance exertion compared to traditional routines, MRT amplifies excess postexercise oxygen consumption (EPOC)—the so-called afterburn effect where calories continue to be consumed postworkout. For those eyeing fat loss, this aspect of MRT is particularly enticing. However, it's essential to understand that MRT, while efficient, doesn't offer easy shortcuts—it demands genuine effort.

Connecting the dots to our earlier conversation brings us to kettlebells. These adaptable instruments shine in the realm of MRT, especially when it comes to performing complexes, combos, and chains—all robust manifestations of MRT, as it happens. Let's dissect these training modalities now, setting the stage for what's to come.

COMPLEXES, COMBOS, AND CHAINS—OH MY!

The primary training tool we'll be using is the kettlebell complex. As mentioned, complexes are a form of metabolic resistance training (MRT); indeed, they are my personal favorite form of MRT, something I gained a reputation for creating through my Kettlebell Workout of the Week and I Bet You Can't Do This Workout series on YouTube (see QR codes). People have consistently told me that my workouts are their favorite "love to hate" training routines. So, take that for what it's worth.

Check This Out

To supplement the content in this book, you'll find the occasional QR code. Often, this will take you to my YouTube channel, where I have years of cataloged exercise demonstrations and kettlebell workouts.

I encourage you to take advantage of this feature, especially since some of the workouts featured in this book have well-produced videos explaining them.

Complexes: At their core, complexes are a series of exercises (typically between two to five) performed in sequence with minimal pauses. Envision carrying out five swings, followed immediately by five squats and then five presses, with the rest period reserved for after the entire set.

Combos: These are akin to complexes but with a slight variation. The sequence involves executing one repetition of each exercise in a cycle, then repeating this loop multiple times before allowing a break. To illustrate: Execute one swing, one squat, and one press in succession, and then cycle through this trio five times before resting.

Chains: This method is a little different. Think of an array of kettlebells sorted by weight (from light to heavy, say) and performing a series of movements (sometimes even the same movement) across the spectrum. Starting with the heaviest kettlebell, you could tackle eight presses, transition to the medium kettlebell, and culminate with the lightest. (Often you want to do the hardest work first and not smoke or tire yourself with lighter sets, which will inhibit how much you can use with the heavier sets.) Known as drop sets, this structure is ideal for muscle building when time is a constraint. Chains also shine in endurance and conditioning scenarios, such as rapidly executing kettlebell swings across varying weights.

These three Cs—complexes, combos, and chains—really represent the core of this book's training methodology. Each fits neatly under the umbrella of MRT, offering a streamlined yet potent strategy for serious, and seriously holistic, physical prowess. Through kettlebells (supplemented occasionally by body-weight exercises), we'll unlock the full potential of these powerful workout techniques.

Still, complexes, combos, and chains aren't the only workout techniques being used, just the dominant ones. We'll incorporate "on the clock" workouts and traditional interval-based workouts, as well. Often, however, these additional methods are variations of the three Cs. Either way, I thought it was worth mentioning.

Okay. Now that we're equipped with the essential background knowledge, let's jump into the core kettlebell exercises that comprise the bulk of the workouts presented in this book. It's important that we get this right.

3

YOUR LIFT LIBRARY

In this chapter, I explain the fundamental kettlebell exercises—the core
ingredients, if you will—that comprise the bulk of workout routines featured in this book. Obvious note: Proper technique is of paramount importance, not just for safety but for performance. Please don't skip this section.

But fear not, this is no tedious tutorial. It's sweaty, hands-on learning.
As each technique unfolds, I'll include a concise workout (lasting between
ten and twenty minutes) that aids in mastering the move while also fueling
calorie burn and strength development. I'm a big fan of workouts that teach
you things, particularly proper exercise technique, and you'll find several of
those here.

Also, a heads-up: While this chapter covers the key kettlebell exercises,
it doesn't encompass every single move presented in this book (there are a
few auxiliary exercises that will be explained as needed when those movements are introduced, with links to demonstrations if further instruction
is required). However, these are the cornerstone lifts. Mastering these

significantly heightens your chances of executing all workouts with flaw-less technique.

And rest assured, you're not left in the lurch. I've curated a playlist on my YouTube channel providing video demonstrations. This collection not only dives deeper into the techniques dis-cussed here but also introduces many of the auxiliary moves sprinkled throughout the workouts of this book. I suggest giving it a watch and bookmarking it for easy access.

SOME OF THOSE "OTHER" EXERCISES

Just to list some of the auxiliary movements you'll find featured in a variety of the workouts to come, which I think are definitely worth taking a minute to watch a video demonstration of: windmills (great for upper-back and shoulder mobility), single-leg deadlifts (awesome for hamstring strength and flexibility), kettlebell lunges (a splendid supplement to the squat), push presses (a usefully explosive press variation), start-stop swings (a swing variation to hammer the quads), and hollow holds (probably my favorite high-impact ab exercise). Again, not an enormous list, and you can find all these demonstrated throughout Pat Flynn social media land, particularly YouTube. Check them out when you get the chance.

THE BIG 6 KETTLEBELL LIFTS AND HOW TO DO THEM

THE KETTLEBELL SWING

We begin with the iconic kettlebell swing. Often considered the bedrock kettlebell exercise, the swing teaches us to hinge at the hips while maintaining proper back posture and lifting a load—a crucial life skill. A certain dashingly clever (and I might add, quite easy on the eyes) young oracle once quipped about the kettlebell swing, describing it as "a violent expression of the hips and one of the few you can get away with outside the bedroom without coming off as impolite or being asked to leave." That oracle? All right, it's me. But jests aside, when you've got the swing down *pat* (aha!), it acts as a springboard to advanced exercises such as cleans and snatches. In fact, flaws in these moves often trace back to defects in the swing, be it a lack of proper hinging or inadequate explosiveness.

In other words, a well-executed swing makes progressing to other exercises slick and efficient whereas bad swings cause a cascade of inefficiencies.

As to the benefits of this exercise, research confirms the kettlebell swing's efficiency, which many already know firsthand: it "simultaneously improve[s] cardiorespiratory fitness, maximum strength, and explosive strength."[4] In everyday language, kettlebell swings help you build strength, endurance, and mobility, all in the same routine. Legendary strength coach Dan John fittingly labels the swing "the fat-burning athlete builder."

Breaking Down the Swing

The kettlebell swing can be distilled into three phases:

1. The setup
2. The hike pass
3. The hip snap

THE SETUP: The setup should have you looking like the center of a football team. I was going to say quarterback, but then I looked it up. The center is the guy who hikes the ball to the wide receiver. Stand a foot-length (that is, the length of one of *your* feet) behind the kettlebell, push your hips back, bend your legs (as seen in the photo), maintain a flat back, and grasp the kettlebell handle with both hands. Your weight should favor your heels, causing the kettlebell to tilt slightly toward you.

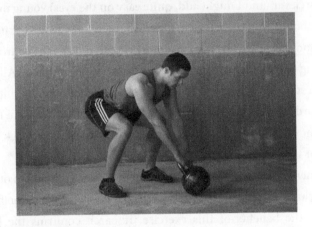

THE HIKE PASS: Engage your armpits, powerfully passing the kettlebell between your legs. Aim to keep the handle above your knees so your back doesn't round. At the base of the hike, your forearms should contact your inner thighs.

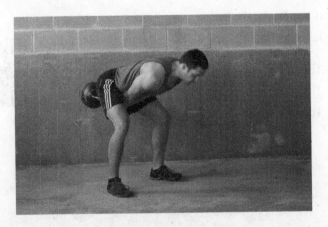

THE HIP SNAP: Visualize performing a broad jump without leaving the ground. Forcefully drive your feet into the ground, slamming your hips forward until you come to a full standing position. The kettlebell should float upward, driven by your hips' power, not your arms.

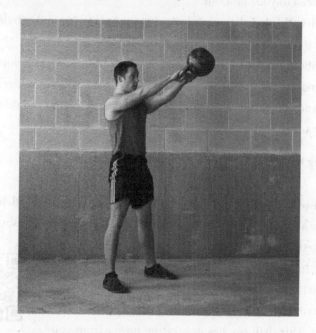

Just a few more notes. First, if the kettlebell lacks "float" or sags on the way up, this means you're not being explosive enough. Recall that the swing is fundamentally a lower-body explosive exercise, not an upper-body shoulder lift. Your hips are the engine, your arms the steering wheel.

Avoid swinging the kettlebell overhead. Ideally, its height should lie between your hips and eyebrows, with the projection of force being more outward than upward. Finally, aid its descent rather than letting gravity do all the work. The more aggressive you are with the downswing, the more explosive you'll be with the upswing, the more strength and power you'll develop, and the more demanding the exercise will be. Just what we want.

Key Technique Notes

Here are three other points to keep in mind while swinging a kettlebell:

- **Back alignment:** Maintain a straight line from the back of your head to your tailbone.
- **Breathing:** Inhale deeply during the backswing and exhale sharply on the upswing, retaining some air.
- **Shoulder position:** Engage your armpit muscles, as if you're holding a $100 bill in there. This should keep your shoulders neutral and "on the shelf"; what we don't want is for the shoulders to get yanked forward.

Facing technical difficulties? Here are two drills:

High-pull deadlift: Start by standing right atop the kettlebell, as if you're about to deadlift it. Now, explode to standing, which should send the kettlebell floating up. Catch it in front of your chest (not with your teeth)—that is, end by holding the kettlebell close to your chest, with your elbows pointed down, not flaring out. Then, slowly lower back down. This drill teaches generating power from your hips. If you find you're bicep curling the kettlebell into position, then try again because that's not right. The arms should be minimally involved, letting all the power come from the lower body.

Start-stop swing: This is a great drill for practicing the beginning and end of each swing. It's simple: Between every swing rep, park the kettlebell back out in front of you. This kills the momentum and forces you to reset and re-engage. It's also important to learn how to safely put the kettlebell down after a set of swings, which this drill reinforces. Every set should finish just how it begins, with the kettlebell out in front, placed with good mechanics (hip hinge, flat back).

The Single-Arm Swing

All right, let's quickly chat about the single-arm swing, a popular variation that pops up all over the workouts in this book. In essence, the single-arm swing is just like the standard (two-hand) kettlebell swing, but—you guessed it—you're only using one hand. (Why one is dubbed "two-hand" swing and the other "single-arm" swing is beyond me; I didn't invent the names, just rolling with them!)

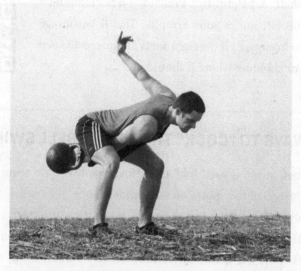

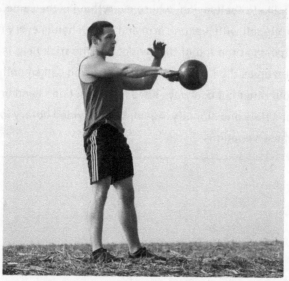

Now, when we talk about the single-arm swing, there are a couple of things to keep in mind:

1. **Torso rotation:** Since you're holding the kettlebell in one arm, it's going to try its hardest to twist your torso. Your job? Don't let it! Keep those shoulders straight and square throughout the swing.

2. **Shoulder position:** The kettlebell is also going to try to yank your shoulder forward. Avoid that by imagining your shoulder is set on a shelf. A helpful tip? Pretend you're clamping a $100 bill under your armpits. That'll encourage you to engage all the right sorts of muscles to keep your shoulder where it should be.

---

2 WAYS TO "COOK" THE KETTLEBELL SWING

The kettlebell swing is excellent as is. However, there are several ways to tweak this exercise to explore an even wider range of benefits. In some of the workouts in this book, we see one such variation, the start-stop swing. As you just saw, this is just where you park the kettlebell between every rep, which really puts the quads to work. Another variation is the single-arm hand-to-hand kettlebell swing, where everything is the same, except you grasp the kettlebell with just one arm and switch hands every rep. Ideally, you switch hands at the top of the swing, and the trick here is to turn the working palm up as the kettlebell elevates, so you can smoothly pass the handle to your other hand, always keeping at least one hand on the bell at all times, for safety and stability. Again, see the video library for a demonstration of these variations.

Workout Time

Okay, workout time. Here is one of my favorite routines for practicing kettlebell swing technique while roasting a bunch of calories.

> **Swings × 30 seconds**
> **Plank × 30 seconds (just hold the top of the push-up position:**
> **flat back, arms straight, abs tight)**
> **Active recovery × 60 seconds (like jump rope)**
> *Continue for 5 to 10 rounds.*

This workout—which my martial arts coach used to call "the old-school lead-in"—is such awesome conditioning. Start with 30 seconds of swings—make them snappy, reminding yourself of proper technique with every rep. Then, hit 30 seconds of plank. This is great to pair with swings because, remember, the top of the swing should feel as if you're in a brief standing plank anyway. Also, it's a classic and always effective core exercise, one you'll see many more times to come. Then, hop up and perform 60 seconds of light, active recovery, either jumping rope or jogging in place. Don't just stand or sit but move lightly as you recover. Repeat this workout for 5 rounds, preferably with no additional rest between. If feeling spirited, perform up to 10 rounds.

Remember, technique takes precedence. Swing into action!

GOBLET SQUAT

Next up: the goblet squat. Another phenomenal lower-body exercise, this one emphasizes the quads more than the hamstrings. Just like the swing is the foundation for more technical exercises like the snatch (we'll get into this later, hold tight!), the goblet squat is the foundation for more technical exercises like the front squat. The more solid the foundation, the more weight you'll be able to lift and the stronger you'll ultimately be.

Goblet squats build strong quads, a stable core, and agile hips. They're a great do-anytime exercise, offering an effective resistance challenge while loosening up stiff body parts. They'll be a regular feature of many of the forthcoming workouts, so take the time to learn the nuances of this exercise.

Anyway, the goblet squat is best learned in contrast to the swing—that is, by practicing them together. Here's why: With the kettlebell swing, your hips go (primarily) back, but in the goblet squat, your hips go (primarily) down. In other words, the swing is all about sending those hips back, almost like aiming to touch that distant wall. In contrast, the goblet squat is all about sending the hips down, as if you're trying to reach your butt to the ground beneath you, pulling yourself straight between your legs.

Moreover, whereas the swing is explosive, the goblet squat is a grind (said differently, if the swing is a firework, the squat is a steady flame). Grinds don't necessarily mean "slow"—they just lack the momentum and snap that are characteristic of moves such as the kettlebell swing and snatch (again, more on this exercise soon). You still want to be continuously powerful with them, but their nature is more even-tempered, and you definitely don't want to "bounce" out of the bottom of a squat. That shows a lack of control and will decrease the benefits you get from the exercise.

Otherwise, goblet squat technique is simple. One reason it's such a useful exercise is because it effectively teaches itself. Simply hold a kettlebell in front of your chest, either by the horns (outside of the handle) or inverted (if that helps your grip). From there, imagine you're pulling yourself between your legs, or pushing your legs apart with your elbows. Your back should stay long and tall, and you should try to remain as upright as possible; in fact, if someone was looking at you from across the room, they should be able to read the front of your shirt. At the bottom, your elbows should come right inside your knees, *not* resting on top. Ideally, your butt should be below your knees, but only go as deep as you can while maintaining a flat back and without your tailbone tucking under or lower back rounding out. Depth will naturally increase over time as you become more accustomed to the exercise.

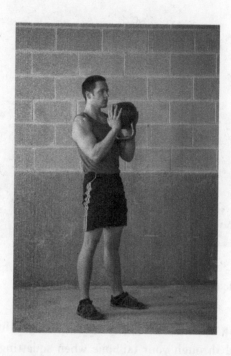

Knee position is important as well. Your knees can and will go forward on the squat. That is fine—despite how often one may hear this, it is a total myth that your knees should never extend out past your toes. Life demands this (try going up a flight of stairs without your knees going over your toes; good luck!), and in fact, your knees are strengthened by deep squats, when done intelligently. What's important is that your knees stay generally *in line* with your toes, meaning your knees don't buckle or bow inward. Keeping your elbows inside your knees will help to prevent this, but ultimately you want them stable on their own, so one thing that can help keep this align-ment is to imagine you're trying to "spread the earth" with your feet, as if you're trying to tear the ground apart. If done right, you should feel the outside of your glutes light up as your knees push more outward. This is a good, strong squatting technique. Use it.

Pause briefly at the bottom of the squat, then stand up, keeping all the mechanics the same. Stand tall at the top, don't lean back. Repeat.

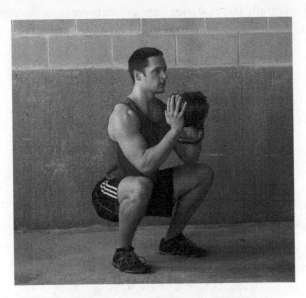

Other technical aspects to keep in mind include:

Flat back: As with the swing, you want a straight line from the back of your head through your tailbone when squatting. However, with the goblet squat, you also want to try to keep your back more vertical, as well as straight. It won't be perfectly vertical—there will always be some lean, which is normal and natural—but try to resist leaning as much as possible.

Breathing match: Also, as with the swing, match breathing to the movement. Inhale to fill your belly with air on the way down, and slowly exhale on the way up. Don't expel all your air—somewhere around 80 percent is enough. You want to keep your belly pressurized as you squat (imagine your lower abdomen region is a balloon; you want to expand it in all directions with air), both for safety and performance, so never completely deflate until the set is done.

SINGLE-ARM SQUAT

The single-arm squat is a simple goblet squat variation where the kettlebell is held in the rack position (which is where you start the military press; see page 34). You'll see this variation featured in quite a number of the workouts in this book, hence why I introduce it now. Technically, everything is the same here as it is with the goblet squat—the only thing that changes is where the kettlebell is held; this position is either the finish of the kettlebell clean or the start of the kettlebell military press, depending on how you look at it. (See those upcoming sections for more detail.)

You can see the single-arm squat demonstrated in this workout complex:

Workout Time

Now for a workout to help reinforce good squatting technique. This workout will pair squats with swings, so you can actively practice the difference in mechanics (remember, for the swing, hips go *back*, for the squat, hips go *down*).

> **Kettlebell swing × 10 reps**
> **Goblet squat × 10 reps**
> **Kettlebell swing × 10 reps**
> **Goblet squat × 8 reps**
> **Kettlebell swing × 10 reps**
> **Goblet squat × 6 reps**
> **Kettlebell swing × 10 reps**
> **Goblet squat × 4 reps**
> **Kettlebell swing × 10 reps**
> **Goblet squat × 2 reps**

As you can see, swing reps stay the same (10) while squat reps ladder from 10 down to 2, by twos. Rest minimally between exercises, as little as you can while keeping good technique. To crank the intensity even more, ladder the squats back up to 10 (i.e., 10 swings, 4 squats, 10 swings, 6 squats, etc.).

MILITARY PRESS

Moving now from fundamental exercises that emphasize the lower body (swings and squats) to exercises that emphasize the upper body, let's discuss the military press.

In terms of bang for buck upper-body strength and muscle-building exercises, the military press—and its more radical cousin the double military press—is about as good as it gets. The rewards are plenty: robust upper-body strength, enhanced muscle definition, spruced up shoulder flexibility and stability, and a sly but potent engagement of the abs. The military press is seriously old-school, a classic strength-building exercise for good reason. It's simple. It's effective.

I mean, what could be simpler than just taking a weight and pressing it overhead? Nevertheless, there are important nuances that can be overlooked even when it comes to exercises that seem perfectly intuitive. Let's cover those now.

Here's how to pull off a proper military press.

The press should begin with the kettlebell in the rack position, which is to say, with the kettlebell resting on the forearm, and with the forearm pinned against the rib cage. Hand and wrist position are important here and easy to miss. You don't want just a neutral wrist, you want a boxer's wrist, where the front two knuckles are lined up with the forearm. This is the strongest, most stable position—the one that is hardest to break. (Hence, it's the position you want when throwing a punch.) When done right, it'll actually look like your hand is tilted slightly forward, but it should feel super strong.

From there, ideally, you want no daylight between the kettlebell and your forearm, and no daylight between your forearm and your body. Fist is below your chin, forearm positioned vertically and pinned against your rib cage. Abs are tight, glutes slightly squeezed, quads engaged. You should feel like you're in a standing plank (that is, abs braced, back flat, glutes squeezed—tight throughout your entire body).

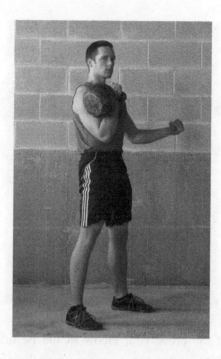

Next step is simple: Begin pressing the weight overhead. However, it's best to imagine you're lifting your elbow to the ceiling, as this tends to keep the shoulder in a more neutral position (you want to avoid shrugging as much as possible). Throughout the entire press, your forearm should remain as vertical as possible. In fact, the best way to find *your* ideal pressing groove is *just* to focus on keeping a vertical forearm—don't let it tilt in, as if you're trying to win an arm-wrestling match.

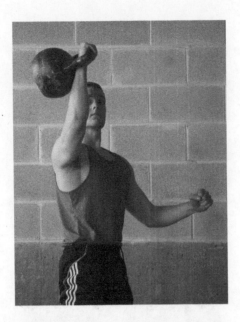

At the top of the press, your elbow should be fully *but not overly* extended, and your bicep should be next to or even slightly behind your ear. That is the full finish.

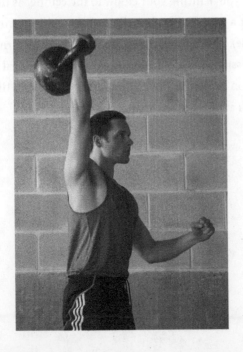

Every press should have the kettlebell come *all the way* back to the rack, with your fist below your chin, forearm against your rib cage.

Finally, all strength in the military press comes from the upper body. Your lower body should be still and locked in place, no bending at the knees or push pressing the weight up. (The push press, where you effectively jump the weight up, is a fine exercise, but it's not *this* exercise.) The military press is all upper-body grind.

Workout Time

Let's practice our pressing technique while building functional strength with the following workout. Go as heavy as you can for each rep range (ideally, use a bell that brings you within 2 reps of technical failure).

> **Military press × 2 reps/side**
> **Kettlebell swing × 15 reps**
> **Military press × 3 reps/side**
> **Kettlebell swing × 15 reps**
> **Military press × 5 reps/side**
> **Kettlebell swing × 15 reps**
> **Military press × 8 reps/side**
> **Kettlebell swing × 15 reps**
> *Two times through.*

This is a seriously great workout to boost functional strength and muscle, especially if you push the intensity as far as you realistically can without compromising technique. The swings between presses give a nice metabolic boost, providing an overall total body workout routine. Again, think of this routine as being as much about practicing technique as it is burning calories, focusing on making each rep as close to perfect as possible.

KETTLEBELL CLEAN

Let's now introduce an essential exercise that bridges the gap between the ground and rack position: the kettlebell clean. To be clear, this exercise is not just a mere transition but a powerful movement in its own right. The kettlebell clean offers a unique combination of power, conditioning, and athletic coordination, engaging both the upper and lower body.

The clean (as will be the case with the snatch) is largely a single-arm kettlebell swing but with a few important tweaks. Whereas the swing is mostly about force production and force reduction, both the clean and the snatch introduce the element of force redirection, and what an important athletic quality that is. In other words, the kettlebell is going to want to go out, but you must direct it back and up into the rack position, which was just introduced with the kettlebell military press, but this also serves as the starting point for other exercises, like the front squat. The clean is how to get there, hence its indispensability.

By itself, the clean targets all the same muscle groups as the swing, but it hits the shoulders and biceps a bit more, since more upper-body engagement is necessary to wrangle the kettlebell into the rack position. Nevertheless, the exercise is still predominantly powered by the lower-body hip snap; the upper body is just there for direction.

Let's break the clean down into the following steps:

1. Hike pass
2. Hip snap
3. Clean into rack

The initial steps of the kettlebell clean should be straightforward enough since they mirror the single-arm swing. Set the kettlebell up no more than a foot in front of you, secure the handle with one arm, then engage your armpit muscles as you push your hips back into a deep hinge. Finally, hike the kettlebell just as you would when performing a single-arm swing to initiate the kettlebell clean.

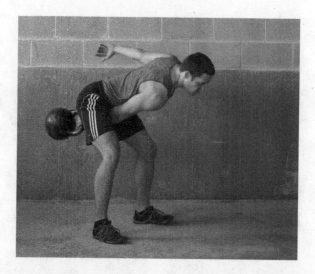

The challenge comes after the hip snap, where you must guide the kettlebell into the rack position. Your objective here is to tame the arc, meaning you must prevent the kettlebell from veering out wildly and then forcefully rebounding toward you, then rebounding into you with great force. Achieving this requires bending the arm, keeping a quiet elbow (ensuring your elbow remains close to your body), and guiding your arm up your center line, reminiscent of zipping up a large coat. When executed correctly, the kettlebell should move closely alongside your body during both the upward and downward phases of the clean, facilitating a smooth transfer onto your forearm.

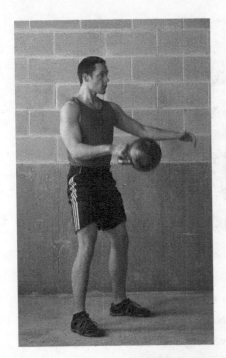
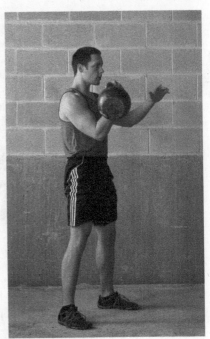
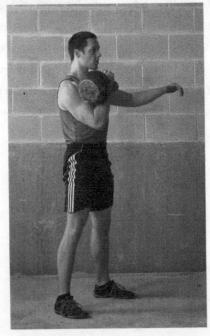

Once the kettlebell is in the rack position, allow it to settle in for just a second. Then, all you're going to do is relax the arm and let the kettlebell fall toward your hips. Timing here is critical because you must move your hips out of the way at the very last second. In fact, you should imagine that you're playing chicken with your zipper—a bold metaphor, but it's effective and ensures you'll instinctively move your hips when necessary. Moving the hips too early can lead to catching the weight with either the lower back or shoulders, or both, which is not optimal. The goal is to use the hips to decelerate the weight, setting up the subsequent rep and transitioning the kettlebell into another backswing.

From there, it's just rinse and repeat.

Let me quickly note one prevalent mistake with the kettlebell clean that often results in bruised forearms and ripped calluses: the tendency to death grip the handle. (This overgripping frequently appears in snatch, as well.) Instinctively, we want to grip the kettlebell firmly to prevent it from inadvertently flying away. Fair enough. However, gripping it too tightly restricts the kettlebell's ability to rotate smoothly onto the forearm. As a result, the kettlebell often slows down, stalls, and then drops violently onto your forearm (rather than smoothly rolling *around* the forearm, as it should), while creating significant strain on the skin of your hands. The solution? Loosen your grip. Hold the kettlebell securely enough to stop it from slipping away but allow enough flexibility for the handle to rotate freely and smoothly during the clean. All this takes practice, of course; it's something you'll ultimately have to get a feel for but is worth being aware of from the start. Your hands and forearms will thank you.

A LITTLE TOUGH LOVE FOR YOUR FOREARMS

Chances are, for much of your life, the back of your forearm has lived a pampered existence, free from the burdensome weight of, well, anything. Enter the kettlebell rack position, and suddenly your forearm is hosting a kettlebell party it never RSVP'd to. It's no wonder that this position often feels, to say the least, a little uncomfortable at first—it's unfamiliar territory. But fear not! With time, just as a martial artist's shin evolves into a formidable force through repeated kicks, your forearm will adapt and toughen. Until that rite of passage, however, prioritize good technique and avoid turning your forearm into a bruise mosaic. A little discomfort is expected, but outright battering? Not on our watch. Bruising isn't good, so let's avoid that. Use common sense and good technique. Gradually amp up the amount of weight or time (or both) to signal your forearms to strengthen without giving them a full-on assault.

Okay, if you're still facing difficulties with the cleaning (don't feel bad, this is one of the more technical exercises; it takes time!), here are two transitional drills that can help.

Single-arm dead clean: Sometimes it's easier to get the feel of the kettlebell swing when the path is more vertical, so one progression people often find useful is the single-arm dead clean. This one is simple. Stand directly atop the kettlebell. Don't hike it back; instead, just deadlift the kettlebell as explosively as possible, so it floats directly up into the rack position. Because the path is now entirely vertical, you should find it easier to transition the kettlebell onto the forearm. Once you begin to feel the groove with the single-arm dead clean, you can immediately move on to the next drill . . .

Reverse kettlebell clean: Either cheat curl (that is, use both arms to curl the kettlebell into the rack position) or dead clean the kettlebell into the rack position. From there, simply relax the arm and "dump" the kettlebell into the hips, moving your hips out of the way at the very last second. Catch the weight with your hips, then park it back at the starting position on the floor. Rinse and repeat. Getting the feel for the clean in reverse often makes it easier to zip it back up. Do so when ready.

Workout Time

This workout combines single-arm cleans with single-arm swings. We'll incrementally increase the cleans but intersperse each set with a single-arm swing. Using swings between cleans effectively reinforces hip hinging, which is important because people often slide into the error of "squatting" their cleans as fatigue sets in.

Here's the routine (start by doing everything on one arm):

> **Single-arm clean × 1 rep**
> **Single-arm swing × 1 rep**
> **Single-arm clean × 2 reps**
> **Single-arm swing × 1 rep**
> **Single-arm clean × 3 reps**
> **Single-arm swing × 1 rep**
> *Switch sides and repeat.*
> *Continue alternating for 15 minutes.*

Remember: Focus on honing your technique with this workout; the calorie burn will naturally follow.

KETTLEBELL SNATCH

Continuing to build upon the foundation of the kettlebell swing, the next fundamental exercise is the kettlebell snatch. The snatch is like the kettlebell clean with a strong element of force redirection—their distinctions lie in the finale of each exercise. While the clean ushers the kettlebell into the rack position, the snatch propels it confidently overhead, necessitating an extra burst of hip-driven power.

The kettlebell snatch really is the epitome of dynamic kettlebell training, seamlessly melding power, precision, and fluidity. Often hailed, somewhat comically, as the czar of kettlebell lifts, the snatch embodies athletic grace. It's not just a lift so much as movement art that demands a subtle blend of explosive power and meticulous control—akin to what martial artists deploy in strikes. The rewards? Never-say-die conditioning, amplified athletic thrust, fortified shoulder stability, a resilient back, and, let's say, "accentuated" biceps. Truly, the snatch is an all-encompassing feat.

Naturally, many of the points covered in the swing and clean immediately carry over to the kettlebell snatch—i.e., power comes from the hips, while the direction comes from the arms and shoulders. We'll break the snatch down into the following steps:

1. Hike pass
2. High pull
3. Punch through

The hike pass is just the same initial start as the kettlebell single-arm swing and clean. Set up about a foot behind the kettlebell, get the armpit muscles engaged, and forcefully hurl the kettlebell into the backswing. From there, jump through your heels, propelling your hips forward. So far, all familiar stuff.

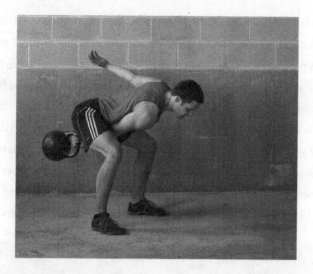

The next step is where things change from both the single-arm swing and single-arm clean. As the kettlebell rides the moment of the hip snap, begin to slacken your elbow. Bend it slightly, while drawing it upward and rearward, as if delivering an elbow strike to some unwanted intruder. Done correctly, this high pull motion should tame the arc of the kettlebell and cause it to arise closely up your center line.

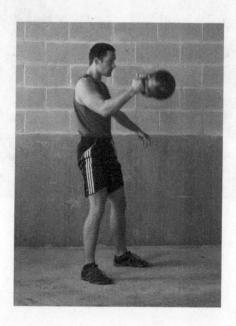

Now, for the most intricate and critical moment: As the kettlebell soars to approximately eyebrow height, there comes a fleeting moment of equilibrium, or a point of levitation, if you will. Seize this moment to swiftly open your hand and energetically punch or thrust (visualize spearheading) your hand through the kettlebell handle, akin to an overly enthusiastic student wanting to be called on in class. When timed correctly, the kettlebell will gracefully roll onto your forearm (not flop over and crash), mirroring the top position of the kettlebell military press. However, remember that you are *not* pressing the kettlebell upward. All power is still coming from the explosive hip snap. The arm merely serves as the guide, not the driving force.

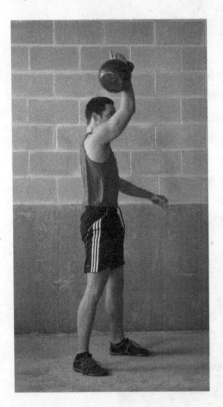 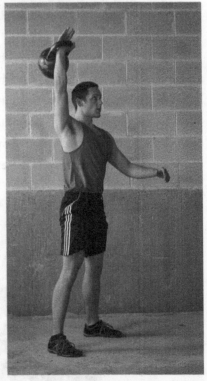

The common mistakes found in the swing and clean are worth keeping in mind with the kettlebell snatch, particularly the point about not over-gripping the kettlebell. Again, keep a grip tight enough to hold on to the kettlebell but not so tight that the handle fails to rotate freely, causing the weight to stall out and flop onto your forearm.

Technical difficulties? No problem. Here are two remedial drills you can use to dial in the kettlebell snatch technique.

1. **High-pull practice:** Quite often it's beneficial to break down complex movements into their more basic components and practice those independently for a while. So, if the snatches are feeling clunky, spend time just practicing the high-pull portion. Start with some single-arm swings and progressively become more aggressive with the high-pull aspect—that is, of drawing your elbow more upward and rearward, trying to feel out for that point of float or levitation. Spear through and finish overhead only when ready.

2. **Drop and catch:** Press a kettlebell overhead into the finish of the snatch position. From here, just practice the movement in reverse but focus on actively throwing the kettlebell into your stomach. This visualization will help you to keep the trajectory of the kettlebell tighter and the path closer to your body. Again, move your hips out of the way at the so-called eleventh hour, catching the weight as you enter into a deep hip hinge. Don't worry about snatching the kettlebell back up just yet. Instead, perform a series of single-arm swings, then set it down. Practicing the movement in reverse will help pattern the groove while sparing your forearms and calluses.

Workout Time

Like the workout focusing on kettlebell clean technique, we'll pad snatch reps with swing and clean reps as reminders for proper hip position and power generation. The workout looks like this:

> **Single-arm swing × 1 rep**
> **Single-arm clean × 1 rep**
> **Single-arm snatch × 1 rep**
> *Switch sides and repeat. Then . . .*
> **Single-arm swing × 1 rep**
> **Single-arm clean × 1 rep**
> **Single-arm snatch × 2 reps**
> *Switch sides and repeat. Then . . .*
> **Single-arm swing × 1 rep**
> **Single-arm clean × 1 rep**
> **Single-arm snatch × 3 reps**

Continue the snatch ladder as high as possible with good technique. If technique fails, revert to just one snatch and begin the ladder anew. Continue for 15 minutes.

Even at the risk of sounding like a broken record, the emphasis on technique can't be overstated: Let this routine serve as a platform to refine and master your snatch technique. Prioritize precision and consistency of each rep. While you'll undoubtedly break a sweat (and likely generate plenty of it), remember that the core objective is technical proficiency.

TURKISH GET UP

The Turkish get up (TGU) is like a carefully choreographed dance with the kettlebell. The only problem is it's just a teensy bit complicated, since the TGU is a composite of many distinct movements. But fear not: I'll simplify this dance into manageable steps for you.

In essence, the TGU is about rising from the ground and then gracefully returning, all while holding a weight—in our case, the trusty kettlebell. Often dubbed the grand odyssey (no idea who named it this) of kettlebell training, the TGU goes beyond mere muscle; it's a master class in spatial awareness and body control. The dividends of mastering this move are many: raw increases of strength, newfound mobility, enhanced stability, and a surefire boost in determination, especially once you begin working heavier sets.

There are many ways to piece apart the Turkish get up, but here's the breakdown I've found most helpful.

1. Setup
2. Roll to elbow
3. Post to hand
4. Bridge to leg sweep
5. Swivel to forward lunge
6. Lunge to stand
7. Reverse!

Let's examine each in turn.

SETUP: First comes the setup. The nuances here are critical because a quality setup ensures a successful finish, while a sloppy setup almost always multiplies mistakes downstream. Here's how to do it. Begin by lying on your side, clutching the kettlebell handle with both hands. Now, hug the kettlebell tight and roll onto your back. Next, stretch out your opposite arm and leg at a 45-degree angle. The leg on the same side as the kettlebell should also be positioned at a 45-degree angle but with the knee bent. Your heel should be relatively close to your butt—not right next to it. (This snow angel position is crucial for strongly getting to the next step). Finally, press the kettlebell straight up, using one or both arms.

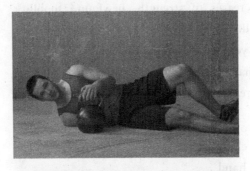

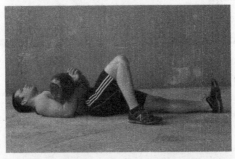

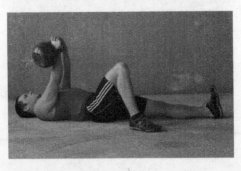

ROLL TO ELBOW: Initiate this stage of the exercise by pressing hard into your planted heel and actively rolling up onto your elbow, all while keeping the kettlebell overhead and your eyes fixed upon it. This phase of the Turkish get up really is a roll and *not* a crunch or sit-up. (In fact, strength coach Dan John once said that if the exercise were called the Turkish roll up, people would probably perform it a lot better and easier.)

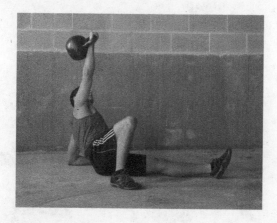

POST TO HAND: The next step is easy. Just straighten out your posted arm, elevating onto your hand (naturally, your fingers will turn and point backward as you transition into this step; let that happen). Keep your shoulders down (think anti-shrug) and eyes on the kettlebell. Your chest should be proud, making it easy for people to read whatever logo or lettering is on your shirt.

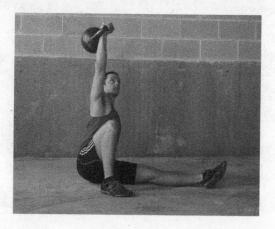

BRIDGE TO LEG SWEEP: Driving through your heel, lift your hips off the ground, creating a bridge. Now, taking advantage of the space you just created between you and the floor, sweep your extended leg back behind you. Ensure your knee aligns with your extended arm, establishing a strong base.

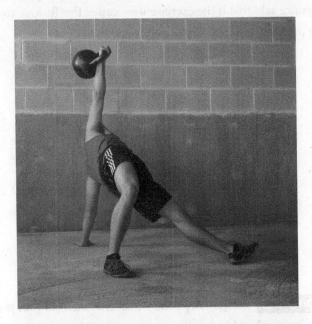

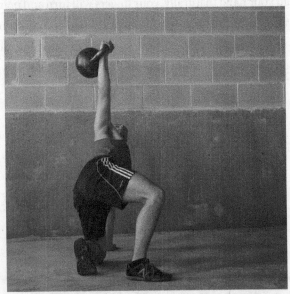

SWIVEL TO FORWARD LUNGE: This is the step almost everyone overlooks. It's subtle but important. Imagine performing the motion of a windshield wiper with your back shin while concurrently pushing your hips back and raising your extended arm. This will naturally lead you into the forward lunge stance, where both knees are now pointed forward and legs are aligned parallel to each other. At this point, the kettlebell should be in the overhead lunge position, with your neck in a relatively neutral position (not too extended) and your eyes either looking slightly up at the kettlebell or straight ahead.

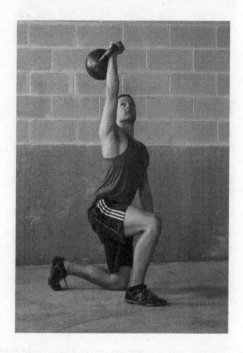

LUNGE TO STAND: The finish is easy. Just complete the lunge to come into a full standing position with the kettlebell head straight overhead, just as it would be positioned in a military press or snatch. Subtle point: Be sure your back toes are planted rather than pointed before lunging, so you can effectively push off your hind leg as you come to standing.

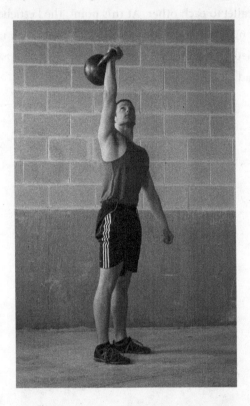

REVERSE: As they say, what goes up must also come down, right? So, to finish the get up, simply reverse each step until you come all the way back to the setup position. To set the kettlebell down, reverse press the kettlebell to your side and roll it back to the ground (again, just reversing how you secured the kettlebell in the first place).

Facing technical difficulties?

If you're struggling to master the Turkish get up, let me offer two ways of approaching it.

Partial get ups: First, just isolate one or two steps of the get up and practice that segment for as much time as you need until it feels completely automatic. Don't worry about getting the entire exercise at once—that's a lot of steps. Maybe just practice the setup and roll to elbow for several days. Then, once those steps feel easy and automatic, add the next one, and continue in this fashion until you've constructed the entire thing. Don't rush!

Reverse get ups: Second, practice the get up in reverse. For whatever reason, many people just seem to have an easier time finding the right positioning throughout the get up when starting from the top down, that is, from the standing lunge position, working backward through each of the steps. My advice? Follow the video linked on page 49 where my buddy Aleks and I work through the get up, step-by-step, in reverse. Once you feel totally comfortable moving through the exercise backward, try starting from the bottom.

2 COMMON TGU MISTAKES

Given that the TGU is a tad more intricate than other exercises, it deserves some extra scrutiny, particularly to address common pitfalls. From my experience, beginners frequently stumble into two consistent mistakes when attempting the TGU.

First, the notorious windshield wiper motion of the back shin often eludes newcomers. During both the ascent and descent of the TGU, forgetting this move leads to limited hip space. The (unfortunate) result? Relying on the lower back to transition into or out of the lunge—a definite no-no!

Secondly, during the descent, there's a tendency to overreach with the free arm, extending it too far behind. Instead of reaching backward, this arm should extend to the side, aiming to land parallel with the stabilized knee (which, remember, you've just adjusted with the aforementioned windshield wiper move).

These admittedly small details are pivotal. They guarantee the optimal alignment during the exercise—a crucial factor as the weight of the kettlebell increases.

Workout Time

The following workout unravels the Turkish get up into its core components, practicing each between a set of two-hand swings. It's a great way to put adequate attention into each step of the TGU while accomplishing a killer workout. Check it out.

> **Kettlebell swing × 10 reps**
> **Setup to elbow roll (RIGHT + LEFT)**
> **Kettlebell swing × 10 reps**
> **Setup to elbow roll + post to hand (RIGHT + LEFT)**
> **Kettlebell swing × 10 reps**
> **Setup to elbow roll + post to hand + bridge to leg sweep**
> *Continue until the entire Turkish get up is constructed.*

Then, start over. See how many *quality* get ups you can construct in 15 to 20 minutes.

DOUBLE YOUR PLEASURE: DOUBLE KETTLEBELL EXERCISES

Aside from the TGU, all the exercises I've detailed so far can be executed with not just one but two kettlebells. To clarify, here is the nomenclature of the double kettlebell variants compared to their single bell equivalents.

Swing → Double swing
Clean → Double clean
Goblet squat → Front squat
Press → Double press
Snatch → Double snatch

Note, while the double snatch is a fine exercise when well executed, I've decided not to prescribe it in any of the forthcoming workouts; it is a bit technical and doesn't offer huge advantages over what we get from double swings and cleans, anyway.

There are benefits to performing exercises with two kettlebells, the obvious one being increased intensity, which can be quite useful when training for strength and muscle. (As you'll see, there are a greater number of double kettlebell exercises in the strength and muscle workout sections than the conditioning and mobility ones.)

There are a few things to keep in mind when transitioning to double kettlebell work. First, you often must adjust your stance to a slightly wider position to accommodate both kettlebells for any of the swinging movements—double swings and cleans. My advice is to go just as wide as you need to accommodate the bells, but no wider. You can maintain this stance for as long as you are performing the swing-based exercises, but I recommend narrowing it to whatever your single kettlebell snatch is when you move to perform double presses or front squats, since you'll then be in a generally stronger and more stable (and safer) position for these exercises. Otherwise, the mechanics of the double kettlebell exercises remain largely, if not entirely, the same as their single bell counterparts.

DOUBLE PRESS

Technical pointer: To avoid redundancy, I won't reiterate all the points about pressing with double pressing, since everything said about the single kettlebell press applies for the double kettlebell press. Rather, I will just emphasize that when pressing two kettlebells overhead, you will want to focus even more intensely on keeping your abs braced and glutes squeezed, since the increased load can cause one to lean back, which is not an ideal position to be in. So, again, imagine you're in a standing plank as you press, with everything tight and engaged as the kettlebells move overhead.

Note: In several of the workouts that follow, you will see *double clean AND press* prescribed. As a quick heads-up, this means to perform a clean between every press. So, double clean and press × 3 reps = double clean, double press, double clean, double press, double clean, double press.

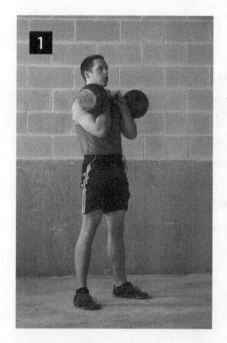
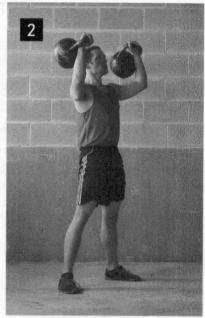
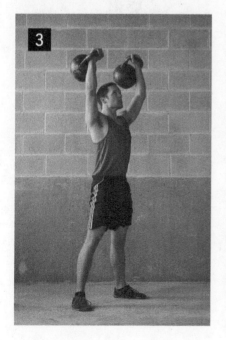
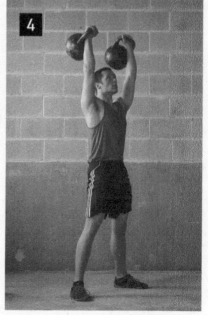

FRONT SQUAT

Technical pointer: Again, everything said about the goblet squat applies to the front squat, with the primary differences simply being load (the amount of weight used) and placement (kettlebells now in the rack position). Since the load is higher with front squats, this can often cause people to round their upper back or collapse their chest inward—sort of the opposite problem one encounters with double pressing, where the tendency is to lean backward. Awareness is the first and best defense: Intensely focus on keeping a long, tall spine throughout the front squat, as if you're trying to reach the top of your head to the ceiling throughout the exercise.

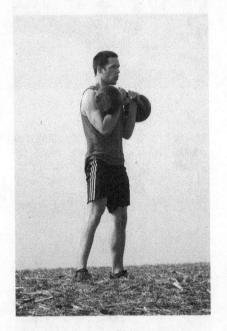
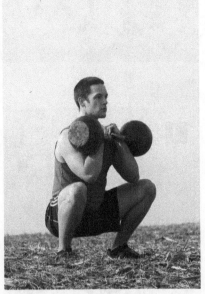

OTHER EXERCISES YOU'LL (SOMETIMES) ENCOUNTER ALONG THE WAY

The exercises above comprise the majority of movements you'll be performing in the workouts to follow. However, there are some stragglers, if you will—I mean, exercises that make an occasional appearance and, because of that, deserve a brief mention and description. Fortunately, most of them are so basic that they are almost impossible to mess up. Nevertheless, I thought a quick rundown of the essential technical points might be helpful. Of course, you can always consult my video playlist for a visual demo. (I also include a direct QR link for each technique.)

PLANK

Perhaps the most basic—but undeniably awesome—body-weight exercise, particularly powerful for building core strength and stability. Here, you're really just holding the top of a push-up position. Key things to keep in mind: flat back, braced abs, squeezed glutes, straight arms. Hand placement should be directly under your shoulders.

HOLLOW HOLD

A deceptively difficult but highly effective direct core exercise. Lie on your back, press your lower back hard into the ground, slightly elevating your hips and shoulders. Brace your abs. You should form into a banana position.

PUSH-UP

Everybody's favorite gym class exercise—still as good as it ever was for building pushing strength and developing chest, shoulder, and arm muscles. Set up in a plank (hands placed under shoulders) and descend by bending the elbows. Ideally, your elbows should be pointed more back than out (flare no more than 45 degrees, but adjust for preference and comfort). Lower with control until your chest about touches the ground, then come back up.

HINDU PUSH-UP

These are really great mobility push-ups, especially for stretching the back and shoulders. The movement essentially combines a forward bend, a backbend, and a traditional push-up. You've likely seen them before, but here's how they work. Get into a standard push-up position. Then, push your butt straight into the air, so your body forms an inverted V shape (for those familiar with yoga poses, this is close to the downward dog position; this is your forward bend). Next, lower your hips and glide your body forward, performing a swooping motion as you bring your chest and hips close to the ground, as if you're trying to dive under a fence. Continue the swooping motion by straightening your arms and arching your back, ending in the backbend (or upward dog) position. Your hips should be low at the point. Look straight ahead or slightly upward at the finish. From here, just push your hips back up to the original position to repeat the exercise. (Note: If you reverse the movement entirely, which is much more difficult, that is called a divebomber push-up.)

SUITCASE CARRY

Deadlift a single kettlebell with one arm and then stand tall while holding the kettlebell off to your side, just like it's a suitcase. The key here is to not bend sideways. Engage your side muscles to stay perfectly straight. A great grip and ab exercise.

FARMER'S CARRY

Essentially the same as the suitcase carry but now with two kettlebells, one on each side. Again, the key is to stand as tall as possible. Don't allow the weight of the kettlebells to cause you to hunch or roll your shoulders forward. Imagine you're pressing the top of your head toward the ceiling as you carry the weight. Another awesome grip and core exercise—great for moving heavy loads and building old-school farm boy strength!

KETTLEBELL HALO

Grab a kettlebell by the horns (sides of the handle) and hold it upside down in front of your chin. From there, simply circle it around your head, drawing a halo. This is a phenomenal shoulder mobilizer and strengthener, and the key to a quality halo is to get your elbows as high up as possible when cir-cling the kettlebell around your head. Importantly, be sure the kettlebell is going around your head and that you are not weaving your head around the kettlebell (meaning your head and neck should remain perfectly still as you perform this exercise).

KETTLEBELL WINDMILL

This exercise really opens up the hips while loosening up the hamstrings and upper back and shoulders. Here's how to do it. Stand with your feet shoulder width apart and press a kettlebell straight over-head, arm fully extended. (You want to keep your arm locked out at all times throughout this exercise.) Next, turn your feet out at a 45-degree angle away from the hand holding the kettlebell (so, if the kettlebell is in your right hand, both feet should point toward your left). Now, begin to push your hips back and to the side (that is, toward the kettlebell side). Keep your eyes on the kettlebell as you naturally begin to hinge, lowering your torso toward the opposite (front) foot. Your free arm should trace down the inside of your front leg, for guidance. Go as low as you can with a *flat* back—that is, only as far as you can by hinging at the hips, *not* bending at your side. (Techni-cally, a proper kettlebell windmill is not like a windmill in yoga, for those familiar with that exercise; in other words, this is not a side bend but rather a combination of hip hinging and thoracic spine rotation.) Pause momen-tarily at the end of your range of motion, then reverse the movement to come back up.

HIP BRIDGE

This simple exercise does a lot to loosen up sticky hips and build strong glutes. Lie on your back, bend your knees, and place your feet flat on the ground, hip width apart. Your arms should be at your sides, palms up (so you resist wanting to press down with your hands). Next, lift your hips by pushing your heels hard into the ground and squeezing your glutes. At the finish, your body should form a straight line from your shoulders to your knees. Hold at the top for one to two seconds, squeezing your glutes very tightly. (Odd but helpful visual: Imagine you're trying to crack an acorn between your cheeks.) Don't overarch your back. Lower fully and with control before starting the next repetition.

KETTLEBELL ROW

One of the fundamental pulling patterns to strengthen your back and biceps. It's very simple: Hinge at the hips with knees slightly bent, hold a kettlebell in one hand, and pull it toward your hip while keeping your back flat and elbow close to your body. Note: This can easily be done with two kettlebells, making this a double row.

4

CHOOSE YOUR GENERALIST
FITNESS ADVENTURE

I n this chapter, I'll outline the various training approaches. While each of these programming schedules shares a broad resemblance, they're crafted to emphasize specific goals, whether that's building strength, muscle, endurance (interchangeably, "conditioning" or "work capacity"), shedding fat, or improving mobility. (There is, undeniably, an overlap between some of these categories, and each of the schedules promotes all the qualities, so again, each of the schedules is promoting a particular emphasis toward your desired outcome. More on that in a minute.)

Before going any further, let me briefly define each of these categories for you and defend the groupings I've decided to use.

For example, when I talk about "strength," I really mean your ability to move against resistance. Strength isn't exactly the same thing as muscle: You can be strong, of course, without being crazy muscular. (Lots of athletes are like this, very strong and powerful yet more wiry in appearance; not every super strong person looks like a bodybuilder!) So, when I talk about "muscle," specifically, I am referring to more focused hypertrophy work (muscle building), where we are actively trying to add weight (lean muscle tissue) to our frame.

Now, this is important: While distinct categories, the relationship between building strength and muscle is still close; however, it's not like you can entirely isolate one from the other. Here's how I like to describe it (this is a common analogy, not original to me but effective): Think of your body as a factory that outputs strength, with your nervous system being the general manager and your muscles being the literal production equipment. Now, one way you can increase strength output is just to increase the efficiency of your nervous system—that is, by training your manager to be more efficient—or, in physiological speak, by increasing neuromuscular efficiency and learning to contract the muscles you have harder. Another way to increase strength is to outright build a bigger factory, which is to say, by putting on more muscle. Both are effective, and you can focus on doing one more than the other, even if focusing on one, to some extent, inevitably gets you some of the other. (You can't build strength without building at least some muscle, and you can't build muscle without getting at least somewhat stronger!)

In other words, depending on how you approach training, some efforts will be more geared toward increasing neuromuscular efficiency and not *as* hypertrophic, whereas other efforts will put more stress and strain on the muscle tissue, encouraging them to grow more. The line demarcating these efforts is not easy to locate, and there is always crossover, but it's generally acknowledged that lower rep strength efforts (five reps or fewer) work more on the neuromuscular efficiency or "manager" side, whereas higher rep sets (eight to fifteen reps) do more for building a bigger factory (more muscle), assuming you are working at a relatively high intensity for each.

Okay, so much for strength and muscle. Moving on.

Conditioning is a general term, often used to describe getting in shape for some specific event, like an MMA fight or triathlon, but for our purposes we're thinking about everyday work capacity, which we defined earlier as the ability to perform and sustain physical activity. This would encompass activities where you could still maintain a conversation with someone while performing (like brisk walking and light jogging) and activities that are far more intense (like sprinting or circuit training) where you could not maintain a conversation. The generalist, of course, should be able to do it all. If nothing else, having stellar work capacity makes you a superstar when it comes to hauling in groceries from the minivan—you'll never get tired doing it! (Sorry, I didn't mean to show off.)

The reason these things are lumped together the way they are is because of their mutual harmony when it comes to various or multiple pursuits. Strength and muscle efforts go well together (especially when conjoined with a calorie surplus), and various conditioning efforts can be quite conducive to fat loss (especially when conjoined with a calorie deficit). That said, muscle and fat loss do not play well together, at least not always at the same time, since one ultimately requires more calories going in, and the other ultimately requires more calories going out. The matter is complicated, of course, since it is possible—and it does often happen—that people build muscle and lose fat during the same stretch of time, but this is often referred to as "newbie gains." As you become more seasoned in your fitness efforts, certain goals can start to compete against each other because of what they require, and the best approach to then achieve the best of all worlds is to begin a process of cycling—that is, of spending certain phases or seasons on building strength and muscle and others on boosting conditioning and losing fat. Over time, as you continue to cycle through these phases or seasons, you start to build a truly impressive physique with remarkable ability. Long story short, while some people can get away, especially if they are just starting out, with getting everything at once, the better, smarter strategy is to focus on just one or two things at a time and pursue them aggressively.

Not to annoy you with endless qualifications (as I proceed to do exactly that), but here's something else. Importantly, while each schedule may emphasize some fitness aspect more than others, no schedule completely neglects any one of those attributes. The schedule emphasizing conditioning still has a good amount of strength and muscle-building efforts, and the schedule emphasizing strength and muscle still has a fair bit of conditioning work. Really, it's just a matter of leaning more in certain directions than others—all these schedules are generalist, working to bring about robust physical preparedness across multiple domains, and each of them utilizes metabolic resistance training (MRT) through kettlebell complexes, combos, and chains.

I've previously emphasized—and it's worth reiterating—irrespective of your specific fitness ambitions, the foundational approach for a generalist remains consistent. This means regular intense weightlifting complemented with a protein-rich diet (perhaps I should have just named this book *Lift Weights, Eat Protein!*). That said, the type and intensity of weightlifting, or in our case, the kettlebell routines, can be adjusted based on what we prioritize and what we enjoy. For instance, if muscle gain tops the list, our sessions might focus more on workouts with higher lifting volume with multiple sets working close to failure, using the big, compound lifts and more double kettlebell work. Conversely, if the goal leans toward conditioning and fat loss (generally, I lump these together because these efforts tend to be mutually reinforcing), we can ease off the lifting volume a bit and introduce more conditioning work with lighter kettlebells. Again, all this can be accomplished through MRT via complexes, combos, and chains; it's mostly just the specifics (which exercises, what order, how many reps) that vary—oh, and the eating plan as well, but we'll discuss that in appendix 2.

Drawing from an analogy that my friend Jim Madden often uses: Good fitness is akin to a Taco Bell meal. It involves using a limited set of proven-effective ingredients and adjusting their proportions to achieve diverse results. Admittedly, referencing Taco Bell in a fitness guide might raise eyebrows, but the essence of the comparison, I hope, is clear. Your training program doesn't necessitate an exhaustive list of exercises or other options. Nevertheless, I understand the yearning for a routine that's both engaging and enjoyable. Hence, I've blended in what I deem "purposeful variety"—enough to keep the routines spirited without veering from our primary objectives.

To keep the journey captivating, we can implement diverse workouts. Following this chapter, you'll encounter quite a comprehensive collection of kettlebell routines. Each, of course, is designed to be seamlessly integrated into the programming schedules we'll discuss shortly—you literally can just grab and go. It's worth noting that you don't *need* to constantly switch up the routine. If a few specific workouts resonate with you, feel free to repeat them throughout your training phase as much as you like (then just switch things up during the next training phase), striving for improvement each time you run the workout—be it in lifting heavier weights or lifting the same amount of weight faster (more sets in the same, or less, time). My mission is to provide you with a solid framework for success while allowing the flexibility to customize your workouts to your liking. I'm aiming for a balanced approach, steering clear of two unhelpful extremes: the overly rigid program that's unrealistic for many and the overly loose and "intuitive" program that lacks effectiveness with regard to efficiently achieving your goals. It's about finding that middle ground.

I present the essential guidelines and give you the freedom to choose the specifics. Isn't that a generous offer?

CHALLENGED BUT SUCCESSFUL

Training should be about patterning success, not setting up for failure. This means constantly approaching your limits without always crossing them to the point of constant failure. It's about challenging yourself to see improvements without ending a workout feeling deflated and demotivated. In essence, it's about pushing boundaries without breaking them.

"Challenged but successful" echoes the overarching intensity approach to strength and muscle-building routines. This involves training up to the brink of technical failure—where you can't perform another rep with proper form—without pushing into absolute failure. That fine line is where you're challenged but still come out successful.

So, let's navigate the process. What follows is a weekly template ("schedule") for which routines are to be performed based on what aspect of fitness you want to pursue most. Each template features four primary training days with an optional day 5. Given that each routine is just twenty minutes, four days of training per week hits the sweet spot, while adding the additional fifth will give a nice little boost without going overboard. On the off days, I recommend walking and stretching. Once you settle on a schedule to begin with, simply fill in each training day with one of the workouts from the collection in the next chapter, which are organized by the categories represented in the training schedules. So, for example, if day 1 prescribes a strength-based routine, then snag a strength-based workout from the workout collection in the next chapter and run that. Then, if day 2 prescribes a conditioning routine, pluck a conditioning workout and run that. It's a breezy, intuitive process.

Let's look at each of the four training schedules now.

FOR STRENGTH

The strength schedule, no surprise, emphasizes—you guessed it—strength workouts! Complemented, of course, with mobility workouts and some (really, just enough) conditioning work. This is an awesome schedule to start with, as it will seriously build a *strong* foundation for everything else. Notice, as well, that for each of the schedules there is an optional day. If you feel energetic and good, run it. Otherwise, omit without guilt.

Day 1: Strength
Day 2: Mobility
Day 3: Strength
Day 4: OFF
Day 5: Conditioning
Day 6: Muscle (optional)
Day 7: OFF

FOR MUSCLE

The muscle schedule effectively just swaps strength and muscle routines, putting a greater emphasis on higher rep hypertrophy efforts. Again, you'll still build strength with this approach, but this schedule would be more suited to people wanting to add a little more weight to their frame, for whatever reason. (I'm sure you could think of some.)

Day 1: Muscle

Day 2: Mobility

Day 3: OFF

Day 4: Muscle

Day 5: Conditioning

Day 6: Strength (optional)

Day 7: OFF

FOR CONDITIONING AND FAT LOSS

Conditioning and fat loss go together because the high-intensity metabolic efforts used for conditioning are superb for cranking the metabolism and searing through calories. As with the other schedules, you'll still get a minimum effective template of strength and muscle and mobility work, but this one is definitely on the sweatier side. Great for people who want to lean out and be able to "go the distance."

Day 1: Conditioning

Day 2: Strength

Day 3: Mobility

Day 4: OFF

Day 5: Conditioning

Day 6: Muscle (optional)

Day 7: OFF

FOR MOBILITY

By mobility, I don't mean this program will make you into a professional contortionist. I really just mean that this schedule will make you feel good and strong in your general movement and is, naturally, a little less intense than the other schedules but still has tough training days. Really and truly, this is a great template to start with, especially if you've been out of the exercise game for a while, or to rotate into when life is busier and more stressful.

Day 1: Mobility
Day 2: Conditioning
Day 3: Strength
Day 4: OFF
Day 5: Mobility
Day 6: Strength or muscle (optional)
Day 7: OFF

So, as you can see, each schedule shares routines with all the others. What changes, ultimately, are just the proportions—that way you're immediately pushed most in the direction of interest. The other critical thing to keep in mind is the eating component, which is discussed in appendix 2. Obviously, if fat loss is a major objective for you, then how you approach eating will be different than if muscle gain is most important, even if you keep the training schedule the same. (However, I recommend starting with the conditioning / fat loss schedule first, if leaning out is what you desire most.)

ON TRAINING CYCLES AND DELOADS

Each training schedule can be run for eight weeks before deloading, then cycling onto something else or running the same training schedule again. By deloading, I mean cutting all the workouts exactly in half—that is, dropping them from twenty to ten minutes. Generally, you can keep intensity (weight) the same; for the deload, we're mostly interested in reducing the overall amount of work you do. If, however, you feel extra recovery is needed, then yes, go lighter. Generally, deloads should last about a week. Sometimes, five days is sufficient, but feel free to extend up to fourteen days or more if you feel you need it.

THE IMPORTANCE OF DELOADING

There's a prevalent notion among (at least the more learned) fitness enthusiasts: If you don't willingly incorporate a deload, you will likely be forced into one because of injury or burnout. So, let's talk about this. Why is deloading important?

1. **Enhanced recovery:** At its core, deloading is about recovery. By temporarily reducing the volume or intensity of your workouts, or both, you offer your body a valuable opportunity to recuperate. This is paramount to ensuring that gains you've been working toward are cemented, or solidified.

2. **Avoidance of overtraining:** Intense, regular exercise can lead to overtraining—a state where your body hasn't had adequate time to recover from the cumulative stress placed upon it. Overtraining can manifest as persistent fatigue, susceptibility to injury, and a consistent decline in overall performance. Oh, and lowered libido.

3. **Microtrauma management:** Intense training induces microtraumas in our muscles, which are tiny tears. These microtraumas are essential for muscle growth and adaptation, but they necessitate healing. Deloading provides the body a window to manage and heal these traumas effectively.

4. **Mental rejuvenation:** Beyond the physical realm, intense training can also be mentally taxing. A deload period, hence, is not just a physiological reprieve but also a psychological one. It offers the opportunity to recharge mentally, ensuring long-term consistency and preventing burnout.

My general recommendation is this: To become a seriously robust generalist, you should try to cycle through each of these training schedules, perhaps even once per year. Since there are fifty-two weeks in a year, and since each training schedule is run for eight weeks, that means you can fit at least six cycles in each year. Try to do that, and just repeat whatever schedule most aligns with whatever goal you care about most. For example, if you really want more strength, then run the strength schedule twice in the same year, whether concurrently or spread out.

Again, I must insist on not making any of this complicated. I just want you to grab workouts and get awesome results, with little thinking involved. My hope is to provide a maximally clear, plug-and-play formula so you can focus your energy on getting the workouts done with gusto. I don't want you to fumble over details that, ultimately, aren't that important. Just settle on a training schedule, insert the relevant workouts (run them with impeccable technique, of course), adhere to the eating guidelines in appendix 2, and watch as your body transforms in the direction you've always wanted it to.

Okay, enough. It's time now to open the quite enormous vault of kettlebell workouts. Are you ready for it? What follows will be the raw material you plug into the training machine to churn out a harder, leaner, more resilient *you*. Let's go!

5
THE MOTHERLODE: 101 KETTLEBELL WORKOUTS

Here it is: the literal motherlode of kettlebell workouts. Just grab your workout and *go*.

As explained in the previous chapter, these minimalist kettlebell routines are meant to be plugged into the programming schedules as you need a routine to fit into each respective training day (strength, muscle, etc.). You can pick randomly if you want, repeat your personal favorites, or just go in order. All are effective options. Go with whatever suits your interests.

Except for some of the mobility routines (which often help promote recovery from the tougher workouts), each workout incorporates some form of metabolic resistance training using kettlebell complexes, combos, and chains. Again, there is a good bit of variety in how each routine is executed, with some routines having you perform a complex at the top of each minute, and other routines just having you cram as much (quality) work as possible into twenty minutes or less. Indeed, every workout, as promised, has a twenty-minute cap—that means no primary workout routine will (or needs to) last longer than twenty minutes. Twenty minutes is more than enough time to get the response we're after, especially if you stay focused and work hard. In fact, shortened workout time seems to invoke Parkinson's Law, where work expands to fill the time allotted to it such that, by compressing our training time, the more intense and focused we tend to be. And that's exactly what we want.

As you'll see, many of the routines have you complete as many sets or rounds as possible, with good technique, in twenty minutes. This leaves two good ways to progress and make your workouts more challenging over time: You can either come back to certain workouts and try to use more weight, or you can try to perform more sets or rounds in the same amount of time. Both are progress and both are worth pursuing at various points.

Otherwise, the workouts are—as promised—simple (though not easy) and time efficient. Mostly, they are comprised of the core kettlebell exercises we took time to study in the previous chapters and their respective double kettlebell counterparts. Occasionally, we may toss in some other supplementary exercise, like push-ups or planks or another kettlebell move entirely. If you're unsure about proper technique for these supplementary exercises, please consult the technique playlist I compiled on my YouTube channel. Moreover, I'll supply notes on several of the workouts whenever I have something either interesting or important to add. But for the most part, I want you to just be able to read them quickly and go!

Finally, let me reiterate the importance of quality technique. Yes, you want to push yourself; as mentioned before, intensity is critical. Still, you don't want to push beyond your limits, just right up to them. Training to the point of complete technical breakdown can lead to injury and reinforce bad habits without necessarily ensuring better or faster progress. In many, but not all, of the workouts, we aim to work close to technical failure—within two-ish reps, in most cases. (Note: This intensity consideration is most applicable to the strength and muscle workouts, less crucial for the conditioning workouts, and completely discouraged for the mobility routines.)

As noted earlier, technical failure is the point where you start noticing a significant decrease in rep quality, such as when you drop in speed or begin making compensatory movements (like leaning during a press or flaring your elbows during push-ups) to complete the reps. Absolute failure, on the other hand, is when the weight becomes immovable for your body, regardless of any compensation or alteration of technique. When it comes to strength and muscle, aim to flirt with technical failure, reaching it directly or within approximately two reps in most cases. Absolute failure is not a concern and should not be pursued—it's unnecessary.

COMMON TERMS

To clarify a couple of prevalent terms you'll encounter in the workouts:

- **Reps:** Short for "repetitions." It indicates how many times you should perform a particular exercise in succession. For instance, "Kettlebell swing × 10 reps" instructs you to execute (like a robot!) the two-hand swing ten times consecutively. Simple, right?
- **AMRAP:** An acronym for "as many rounds as possible." When you spot "AMRAP 20 minutes" (a common occurrence given that the workouts typically last twenty minutes or less), this just means that you should aim to complete as many rounds as feasible of whatever is prescribed *with good form* in twenty minutes.

STRENGTH WORKOUTS

Armor Building (Single Bell)

The idea of armor building comes from strength coach Dan John. He uses this complex to "harden" his athletes.

Single-arm clean × 2 reps
Single-arm press × 1 rep
Single-arm squat × 3 reps
Switch sides and repeat.

Prescription: AMRAP 20 minutes.
Weight: Use a weight that is between your 2- and 5-rep pressing max.

Armor Building (Double Bell)

Really, same as the previous workout, but now with the increased intensity of two kettlebells.

Double clean	×	2 reps
Double military press	×	1 rep
Front squat	×	3 reps

Prescription: AMRAP 20 minutes.

Weight: Use a weight that is between your 2- and 5-rep pressing max.

Get Down!

This is a neat workout because it allows you to work your way down to the ground and then back up again, after being a bit fatigued. An important life skill, to be sure.

Single-arm clean	×	3 reps
Single-arm push press	×	2 reps
Reverse Turkish get up	×	1 rep

Switch sides and repeat.

Prescription: AMRAP 20 minutes.

Weight: Use a weight that is between your 2- and 5-rep pressing max.

Traveling Twos (Single Bell)

Imagine this workout is like a snake with a mouse traveling through it, since a lump of reps moves through the complex each round.

Single-arm swing	×	2 reps
Single-arm clean	×	1 rep
Single-arm squat	×	1 rep
Single-arm swing	×	1 rep
Single-arm clean	×	2 reps
Single-arm squat	×	1 rep
Single-arm swing	×	1 rep
Single-arm clean	×	1 rep
Single-arm squat	×	2 reps

Switch sides and repeat.

Prescription: AMRAP 20 minutes.
Weight: Use a weight that is between your 2- and 5-rep pressing max.

Traveling Twos (Double Bell)

Same concept as the previous workout—now we're just doubling up the kettlebells.

Double kettlebell swing	×	2 reps
Double clean	×	1 rep
Front squat	×	1 rep
Double kettlebell swing	×	1 rep
Double clean	×	2 reps
Front squat	×	1 rep
Double kettlebell swing	×	1 rep
Double clean	×	1 rep
Front squat	×	2 reps

Prescription: AMRAP 20 minutes.

Weight: Use a weight that is between your 2- and 5-rep pressing max.

Press and Swing Chain

Note: *Chains follow a similar pattern: You line up a string of bells and then perform an exercise or collection of exercises at each one. They are a tremendous way to build volume—that is, get a lot of quality reps in—in a fairly short time.*

Line up three kettlebells (one light, one medium, and one heavy, relative to pressing). At each bell (it doesn't matter which one you start with, since you'll be cycling through continuously), complete:

Single-arm press　×　2 reps
Single-arm swing　×　5 reps
Switch arms at each bell.

Prescription: Cycle through the chain as many times as possible in 20 minutes.
Weight: The heavy weight should be between your 3- and 5-rep pressing max.

Row and Squat Chain

Line up three kettlebells (one light, one medium, and one heavy, relative to rowing). At each bell, complete:

Single-arm row × 2 reps
Goblet squat × 5 reps
Switch rowing arms at each bell.

Prescription: Cycle through the chain as many times as possible in 20 minutes.

Weight: The heavy weight should be between your 3- and 5-rep rowing max.

Snatch to (Reverse) Get Up

Okay, this one is a little different because you will actually begin your Turkish get up from the finish of the kettlebell snatch (standing up with the kettlebell overhead), effectively performing a Turkish get down. It's an awesome flow!

Snatch to reverse Turkish get up × 1 rep (start the TGU from the top, work down, then back to standing)
Switch sides and repeat.
Snatch × 2 reps + reverse Turkish get up × 1 rep
Switch sides and repeat.
Snatch × 3 reps + reverse Turkish get up × 1 rep
Switch sides and repeat.
Continue to add snatch reps until you reach 5 snatches each side.
    Then, start over and begin the sequence again.

Prescription: Run up the ladder as many times as possible in 20 minutes.
Weight: Use a weight that is around your 5-rep pressing max.

Strength O'clock

Note: *"Every minute on the minute" routines are one of my favorite, go-to minimalist training options. They work like this. At the top of each minute, you'll perform some prescribed exercise for some prescribed number of reps. Get those reps done as quickly as possible with good technique. Then, you have the rest of the minute to rest. The goal of these workouts is to stay on the clock—that is, not to take any additional rest (unless, of course, you absolutely need to in order to maintain proper technique; commonsense rules always apply!).*

Every minute on the minute:

Minute 1: **Double clean and press***   ×   **3 reps**
Minute 2: **Front squat**   ×   **2 reps**
Minute 3: **Double clean and press**   ×   **2 reps**
Minute 4: **Front squat**   ×   **5 reps**

Prescription: Repeat for 20 minutes. Your goal is to begin each set at the top of every minute (obviously, take additional rest if form begins to fail).
Weight: Use a weight that is around your 5-rep double pressing max.

   *Reminder: Whenever you see *double clean AND press*, this means to perform a clean between every press. So, double clean and press × 3 reps = double clean, double press, double clean, double press, double clean, double press.

Strong on the Minute

Every minute on the minute:

Minute 1: Single-arm military press × 2 reps + single-arm clean
   × 5 reps + single-arm squat × 3 reps (RIGHT)
Minute 2: Single-arm military press × 2 reps + single-arm clean
   × 5 reps + single-arm squat × 3 reps (LEFT)

Prescription: Try to stay on the clock for 15 to 20 minutes.
Weight: Use a weight that is around your 5-rep pressing max.

Snatch Time

Every minute on the minute:

Minute 1: Snatch × 3 reps + single-arm military press × 3 reps
   (from the top of the final snatch) (RIGHT)
Minute 2: Snatch × 3 reps + single-arm military press × 3 reps
   (from the top of the final snatch) (LEFT)

Prescription: Try to stay on the clock for 15 to 20 minutes.
Weight: Use a weight that is between your 3- and 5-rep pressing max.

Traveling Fives (Single Bell)

*Remember Traveling Twos? Well, this is Traveling Fives.
Can you guess what the difference might be?*

Single-arm clean   × **5 reps**
Single-arm press   × **1 rep**
Single-arm squat   × **1 rep**
Switch sides and repeat. Then . . .
Single-arm clean   × **1 rep**
Single-arm press   × **5 reps**
Single-arm squat   × **1 rep**
Switch sides and repeat. Then . . .
Single-arm clean   × **1 rep**
Single-arm press   × **1 rep**
Single-arm squat   × **5 reps**

Prescription: AMRAP 20 minutes.

Weight: Use a weight that is between your 5- and 8-rep pressing max.

Traveling Fives (Double Bell)

Double clean	×	5 reps
Double military press	×	1 rep
Front squat	×	1 rep
Double clean	×	1 rep
Double military press	×	5 reps
Front squat	×	1 rep
Double clean	×	1 rep
Double military press	×	1 rep
Front squat	×	5 reps

Prescription: AMRAP 20 minutes.

Weight: Use a weight that is between your 5- and 8-rep double pressing max.

Day on the Farm

Note: *Here you'll see the farmer's carry make an appearance. This exercise is so simple it's almost impossible to do wrong (just the way I like it!)—you literally just pick up two kettlebells (deadlift them) and hold them to your side, as you would your luggage. Keep a long, tall spine, maintain proper posture, and go for a walk. Tremendous exercise for building grip strength and sneakily hitting the abs, as well.*

Double clean and press	×	1 rep
Farmer's carry	×	20 seconds
Front squat	×	1 rep
Plank	×	20 seconds
Double clean and press	×	3 reps
Farmer's carry	×	20 seconds
Front squat	×	3 reps
Plank	×	20 seconds
Double clean and press	×	5 reps
Farmer's carry	×	20 seconds
Front squat	×	5 reps
Plank	×	20 seconds

Prescription: AMRAP 20 minutes.

Weight: Use a weight that is between your 5- and 8-rep pressing max.

Just the Basics 1

This is definitely one of those OG kettlebell workouts—just swings and get ups!

Single-arm swing × **10 reps**
Turkish get up × **10 reps**
Switch sides and repeat.

Prescription: AMRAP 15 to 20 minutes.
Weight: Use a weight that is around your 3-rep TGU max.

Just the Basics 2

Another OG kettlebell workout. In particular, this should allow you to press a fairly heavy load, as you climb from 1 to 5 reps, with a dash of swings around each set of presses for added conditioning. Simple, but super effective. I love this routine.

Kettlebell swing	×	10 reps
Single-arm military press	×	1 rep/side
Kettlebell swing	×	10 reps
Single-arm military press	×	2 reps/side
Kettlebell swing	×	10 reps
Single-arm military press	×	3 reps/side
Kettlebell swing	×	10 reps
Single-arm military press	×	4 reps/side
Kettlebell swing	×	10 reps
Single-arm military press	×	5 reps/side

Prescription: AMRAP 20 minutes.

Weight: Use a weight that is between your 5- and 7-rep pressing max.

Just the Basics 3

*Workouts like these are—for lack of a better word—fun.
One exercise escalates in reps each round, while the other
remains the same. Really, it's just a slick way to add extra intensity without
making things completely undoable.*

Front squat	×	2 reps
Snatch	×	2 reps/side
Front squat	×	3 reps
Snatch	×	2 reps/side
Front squat	×	5 reps
Snatch	×	2 reps/side

Prescription: AMRAP 20 minutes.

Weight: Use a weight that is between your 5- and 7-rep squatting
max for the squats and a weight that is between your 5- and 7-rep
snatching max for the snatches.

Twos Up

Single-arm swing × 2 reps/side
Single-arm clean × 2 reps/side
Single-arm press × 2 reps/side
Single-arm squat × 2 reps/side

Prescription: AMRAP 15 to 20 minutes.

Weight: Use a weight that is between your 3- and 5-rep pressing max.

Easy as 1, 2, 3?

Note: *Because the reps are quite low with this routine, you really want to make sure you're opting for a sufficiently challenging weight.*

Single-arm press × 1 rep/side
Single-arm squat × 1 rep/side
Single-arm press × 2 reps/side
Single-arm squat × 1 rep/side
Single-arm press × 3 reps/side
Single-arm squat × 1 rep/side

Prescription: AMRAP 15 to 20 minutes.

Weight: Use a weight that is between your 3- and 5-rep pressing max.

Twister

*Named after my favorite "63 percent on the Tomatometer"
movie on Rotten Tomatoes.*

Single-arm swing (or clean or	
snatch; take your pick!)	× **8 reps**
Single-arm squat	× **5 reps**
Single-arm press	× **2 reps**
Single-arm row	× **3 reps**

Switch sides and repeat.

Prescription: AMRAP 20 minutes.

Weight: Use a weight that is between your 5- and 7-rep pressing max.

Get Up Medley

This one—which originally comes from my friend Jim Madden—is loads of . . . "fun"? Sure, we'll go with that. Let's quickly cover some detail. Really, you're just going to start performing Turkish get ups with a light, comfortable weight, and then work to increase the weight until you feel you've reached a significant challenge for just 1 rep. Be safe, of course, but work up to a relatively high intensity.

Note: *Start with your lightest bell, jumping up a bell size (or two) every set or every other set, eventually working up to what feels like a solid working weight for the day. Your goal is to perform at least 5 sets with the heaviest weight you can use safely and confidently within 20 minutes.*

Turkish get up × 1 rep
Switch sides and repeat, jumping up a bell size or two at every other set.

Prescription: Perform sets for 20 minutes, and get at least 5 sets with the heaviest safe weight within that time.
Weight: The heavy bell should be between your 2- and 3-rep TGU max. Men, shoot for 24 to 32 kg; women, 12 to 20 kg.

Prometheus

*This one will definitely make you feel the burn. It's been
something of a cult favorite among my kettlebell followers
on YouTube. Also, you can check out a more fully developed program around
this workout on my Kettlebell Quickies channel:*

Double clean and press	×	**5 reps**
Front squat	×	**5 reps**

Prescription: AMRAP 20 minutes.
Weight: Use a weight that is between your 7- and 10-rep pressing
max.

High Five

*Five reps of five big moves (I count clean and press as two
moves), finished with 1 rep of the Turkish get up at the end.
What more could you want? What more do you need?*

Double swing	×	5 reps
Double clean and press	×	5 reps
Front squat	×	5 reps
Double row	×	5 reps
Turkish get up	×	1 rep/side

Prescription: AMRAP 20 minutes.

Weight: Use a weight that is between your 8- and 12-rep pressing max.

High Power

Single-arm swing	×	5 reps/side
Single-arm press	×	2 reps/side
Single-arm squat	×	3 reps/side

Prescription: AMRAP 20 minutes.

Weight: Use a weight that is between your 3- and 5-rep pressing max.

Heavy Walk

Note: *If you don't have the space to walk the weight around for this workout, then march in place. For added intensity, carry the weight up and down a small hill.*

Front squat	×	**5 reps**
Farmer's carry	×	**20 seconds**
Double push press	×	**3 reps**
Farmer's carry	×	**20 seconds**

Prescription: AMRAP 20 minutes.

Weight: Use a weight that is between your 5- and 7-rep push press max.

Press!

Note: *Here you'll see the suitcase carry. This is the same as the farmer's carry, except instead of two kettlebells, now you're holding only one.*

Single-arm military press	×	**4 reps/side**
Suitcase carry	×	**10 seconds/side**
Kettlebell swing	×	**10 reps**

Prescription: AMRAP 20 minutes.

Weight: Use a weight that is between your 5- and 7-rep pressing max.

MUSCLE
WORKOUTS

Ol' Fibonacci (Lower-Body Emphasis)

WORKOUT

1

*For those who always thought math class was useless,
think again! The Fibonacci sequence is a series of numbers
where each number is the sum of the two preceding. When done in reverse
order, starting at eight, it makes for the perfect muscle-building sequence,
especially when run with big, compound exercises.*

Double clean	×	**8 reps**
Front squat	×	**5 reps**
Double clean	×	**5 reps**
Front squat	×	**3 reps**
Double clean	×	**3 reps**
Front squat	×	**2 reps**
Double clean	×	**2 reps**
Front squat	×	**1 rep**

Prescription: Perform this entire sequence without setting the kettlebells down. AMRAP 20 minutes.

Weight: Use a weight that is between your 10- and 15-rep squatting max.

Ol' Fibonacci (Upper-Body Emphasis)

Same reverse Fibonacci sequence, different selection of exercises.

Double clean	×	8 reps
Double military press	×	5 reps
Double clean	×	5 reps
Double military press	×	3 reps
Double clean	×	3 reps
Double military press	×	2 reps
Double clean	×	2 reps
Double military press	×	1 rep

Prescription: Perform this entire sequence without setting the kettlebells down. AMRAP 20 minutes.

Weight: Use a weight that is between your 10- and 15-rep pressing max.

Muscle Minute

The neat thing about this EMOM routine is that the staggered rep sequences should allow you to stay on the clock while maintaining a high intensity throughout.

Every minute on the minute:

Minute 1: Double press   ×   8 reps
Minute 2: Front squat   ×   2 reps
Minute 3: Double press   ×   2 reps
Minute 4: Front squat   ×   8 reps

Prescription: AMRAP 20 minutes.

Weight: Use a weight that is between your 10- and 12-rep pressing max.

Old-School Push and Pull

Just a classic but deadly effective push/pull routine for you, with a little something for the abs thrown in.

Single-arm press	×	8 reps/side
Push-up	×	20 seconds
Single-arm row	×	8 reps/side
Plank	×	20 seconds

Prescription: AMRAP 20 minutes.

Weight: Use a weight that is between your 12- and 15-rep pressing max.

Push and Squat Combo (Single Bell)

Single-arm military press × 6 reps
Single-arm squat   × 12 reps
Switch sides and repeat.

Prescription: AMRAP 20 minutes.

Weight: Use a weight that is between your 8- and 12-rep pressing max.

Push and Squat Combo (Double Bell)

Double military press × 6 reps
Front squat   × 12 reps

Prescription: AMRAP 20 minutes.

Weight: Use a weight that is between your 8- and 12-rep pressing max.

Pull and Hinge Combo (Single Bell)

Single-arm row   × **6 reps**
Single-arm clean   × **12 reps**
Switch sides and repeat.

Prescription: AMRAP 20 minutes.

Weight: Use a weight that is between your 8- and 12-rep rowing max.

Pull and Hinge Combo (Double Bell)

Double row   × **6 reps**
Double clean   × **12 reps**

Prescription: AMRAP 20 minutes.

Weight: Use a weight that is between your 8- and 12-rep rowing max.

Total Body Crush

Note: *This is an escalating rep sequence, which means each round increases the number of times you perform each exercise. It's quite intense!*

Double clean	×	4 reps
Double military press	×	4 reps
Front squat	×	4 reps
Farmer's carry	×	20 seconds
Double clean	×	6 reps
Double military press	×	6 reps
Front squat	×	6 reps
Farmer's carry	×	40 seconds
Double clean	×	8 reps
Double military press	×	8 reps
Front squat	×	8 reps
Farmer's carry	×	60 seconds

Prescription: Run the sequence twice or AMRAP 20 minutes.

Weight: Use a weight that is between your 10- and 12-rep pressing max.

The Great Push Press and Front Squat Pyramid

Double push press	×	1 rep
Front squat	×	1 rep
Double push press	×	2 reps
Front squat	×	2 reps
Double push press	×	3 reps
Front squat	×	3 reps

Continue increasing the number of reps per set until you reach 10 reps of each exercise. Time and energy permitting, work your way back down to 1 rep.

Prescription: Complete as much of the pyramid as possible in 20 minutes.

Weight: Use a weight that is between your 12- and 15-rep double push press max.

The Great Snatch and Goblet Squat Pyramid

Snatch	×	1 rep/side
Goblet squat	×	1 rep
Snatch	×	2 reps/side
Goblet squat	×	2 reps
Snatch	×	3 reps/side
Goblet squat	×	3 reps

Continue increasing the number of reps per set until you reach 10 reps of each exercise. Time and energy permitting, work your way back down to 1 rep.

Prescription: Complete as much of the pyramid as possible in 20 minutes.
Weight: Use a weight that is between your 12- and 15-rep snatching max.

Kettlebell Cyclone

Here's a good example of a kettlebell cycle, where you perform 1 rep of each exercise at a time but cycle through the sequence multiple times before setting the kettlebell down. It's a great way to accumulate volume for each respective muscle group, while accomplishing a truly total body workout.

Double clean × **1 rep**
Front squat × **1 rep**
Push-up × **1 rep**
Continue for 6 cycles before resting.

Prescription: AMRAP 20 minutes.

Weight: Use a weight that is between your 8- and 10-rep squatting max.

Garbage Cookie

Remember those cookies with, like, way too much stuff in them, but somehow, they still turn out amazing? Here's the workout equivalent.

Double row	×	**5 reps**
Double military press	×	**5 reps**
Front squat	×	**10 reps**
Double kettlebell swing	×	**20 reps**

Prescription: AMRAP 20 minutes.

Weight: Use a weight that is between your 8- and 12-rep pressing max.

All Bases Covered

Every minute on the minute:

Minute 1: Double kettlebell swing × **10 reps**
Minute 2: Front squat × **5 reps**
Minute 3: Push-up × **3 reps**
Minute 4: Double row × **2 reps**

Prescription: AMRAP 20 minutes.
Weight: Use a weight that is between your 10- and 15-rep squatting max.

Reverse Order

Every minute on the minute:

Minute 1: Double kettlebell swing × **2 reps**
Minute 2: Front squat × **3 reps**
Minute 3: Push-up × **5 reps**
Minute 4: Double row × **10 reps**

Prescription: AMRAP 20 minutes.

Weight: Use a weight that is between your 10- and 15-rep rowing max.

Prometheus Returns

Note: *The volume (amount of total work) you perform here is quite high. The temptation will be to go lighter to compensate. Don't!*

Double clean and press	×	**10 reps**
Front squat	×	**10 reps**

Prescription: AMRAP 20 minutes.

Weight: Use a weight that is between your 12- and 15-rep pressing max.

The Octopus

Obviously, this workout will involve 8 reps of each exercise, given the name. I wonder what we could follow this up with?

Double kettlebell swing	×	8 reps
Front squat	×	8 reps
Push-up	×	8 reps
Double clean	×	8 reps
Double military press	×	8 reps
Double row	×	8 reps

Prescription: AMRAP 20 minutes.

Weight: Use a weight that is between your 12- and 15-rep pressing max.

The Squid

N.B.: Brilliant.

Single-arm military press	×	10 reps/side
Reverse lunge	×	10 reps/side
Single-arm swing	×	10 reps/side

Prescription: AMRAP 20 minutes.

Weight: Use a weight that is between your 12- and 15-rep pressing max.

This One Stings . . .

Goblet squat	×	10 reps
Start-stop kettlebell swing	×	10 reps
Deadlift	×	10 reps

Prescription: AMRAP 20 minutes.

Weight: Use a weight that is between your 15- and 20-rep squatting max.

Lower-Body Pain Chain

Line up three kettlebells (heavy, medium, light).

At each kettlebell, perform:

Goblet squat   × 8 reps
Kettlebell swing × 5 reps
Push-up   × 3 reps

Don't rest until you've run the entire chain (effectively completing a huge drop set).

Prescription: AMRAP 20 minutes.

Weight: The heavy weight should be between your 15- and 20-rep squatting max.

Lower-Body Pain Chain DOUBLED

Line up three *sets* of kettlebells (heavy, medium, light).

At each set of kettlebells, perform:

Front squat   ×   8 reps
Double clean   ×   5 reps
Push-up   ×   3 reps
Don't rest until you've run through the entire chain.

Prescription: AMRAP 20 minutes.

Weight: The heavy set should be between your 12- and 15-rep squatting max.

Upper-Body Pain Chain

Line up three kettlebells (heavy, medium, light).
At each kettlebell, perform:

Single-arm military press	×	8 reps/side
Single-arm row	×	5 reps/side
Push-up	×	3 reps

Don't rest until you've run the entire chain (effectively completing a huge drop set).

Prescription: AMRAP 20 minutes.

Weight: The heavy bell should be between your 12- and 15-rep pressing max.

Upper-Body Pain Chain DOUBLED

Line up three *sets* of kettlebells (heavy, medium, light).
At each set of kettlebells, perform:

Double military press	×	8 reps
Double row	×	5 reps
Push-up	×	3 reps

Don't rest until you've run through the entire chain.

Prescription: AMRAP 20 minutes.

Weight: The heavy set should be between your 12- and 15-rep pressing max.

Is This Mean?

Note: *Again, a lot of volume, so the temptation will be to set the kettlebells down before finishing the sequence. Really try not to!*

Double press	×	10 reps
Front squat	×	10 reps
Double swing	×	10 reps
Double row	×	10 reps

Prescription: AMRAP 20 minutes.

Weight: Use a weight that is between your 12- and 15-rep pressing max.

The Eagle

Here's another internet-famous workout originally devised by strength coach Dan John.

Front squat × **8 reps**
Farmer's carry × **20 seconds**

Prescription: AMRAP 20 minutes.
Weight: Men use two 20- to 28-kg kettlebells; women, two 12- to 20-kg bells.

The Beagle

Note: *Rack hold refers to the beginning position of the military press and front squat when used as an exercise in itself—specifically where the kettlebell (or kettlebells, if we're specifying doubles) is held in the rack position for some period of time. Your job is to keep the abs braced, glutes squeezed, and stay tall—don't let the weight of the kettlebell(s) cause you to lean back. You should feel like you're in a standing plank.*

Double press	×	**8 reps**
Double rack hold	×	**20 seconds**
Front squat	×	**2 reps**

Prescription: AMRAP 20 minutes.

Weight: Use a weight that is between your 12- and 15-rep pressing max.

You're Gonna Feel This One!

Single-arm clean   ×   8 reps/side
Single-arm squat   ×   8 reps/side
Single-arm swing   ×   8 reps/side

> **Prescription:** AMRAP 20 minutes.
> **Weight:** Men use 20 to 28 kg; women, 12 to 20 kg.

Level Changes

Note: *The concept of level changes refers simply to getting up and off the ground or, more specifically, going from perpendicular to horizontal positions. Life often has us working at different angles, so it's good that our training (at least occasionally) reflects that.*

Every minute on the minute:

Minute 1: Double clean and press   ×   **8 reps**
Minute 2: Plank   ×   **20 seconds**
Minute 3: Front squat   ×   **8 reps**
Minute 4: Hollow hold   ×   **20 seconds**
Minute 5: Rest

> **Prescription:** AMRAP 20 minutes.
> **Weight:** Use a weight that is between your 12- and 15-rep pressing max.

Simple but Not Easy!

Single-arm swing	×	10 reps/side
Single-arm press	×	5 reps/side
Single-arm squat	×	10 reps/side
Lunge	×	10 reps/side

Prescription: AMRAP 20 minutes.

Weight: Use a weight that is between your 7- and 10-rep pressing max.

CONDITIONING WORKOUTS

High Voltage

This routine has long been my go-to conditioning workout when crunched for time. It never fails to produce the perfect workout.

Single-arm swing	×	**5 reps**
Single-arm clean and press	×	**5 reps**
Single-arm snatch	×	**5 reps**
Single-arm squat	×	**5 reps**
Push-up	×	**5 reps**

Switch sides and repeat.

Prescription: AMRAP 20 minutes.

Weight: Use a weight that is between your 10- and 15-rep pressing max.

The 9-Minute Workout (Really, 18-Minute Workout)

WORKOUT
2

Note: *This is another one of my internet-famous work-out routines, known for its nasty attitude. The idea is to perform a string of exercises, for 60 seconds each, to form a full kettlebell sequence that is 9 minutes in length—in other words, to work for 9 minutes without taking a rest or setting the bell down. Ready for it?*

Since there are some different exercises thrown into the mix here, I highly recommend watching my video demonstration of my 9-Minute Workout.

Single-arm swing	×	30 seconds/side
Single-arm clean and press	×	30 seconds/side
Single-arm snatch	×	30 seconds/side
Single-arm push press	×	30 seconds/side
Reverse lunge	×	30 seconds/side
Single-leg deadlift	×	30 seconds/side
Swing burpee (swing, sprawl to the side, push-up; repeat)	×	30 seconds/side
Plank	×	60 seconds
Thruster (deep squat into overhead press, using momentum from the squat to lift the kettlebell overhead)	×	30 seconds/side

Prescription: Perform the workout twice, resting 2 minutes between each round to keep the entire routine to 20 minutes.
Weight: Men use 16 to 20 kg; women, 8 to 12 kg.

Kickin' It Old School

Cool thing: *You can often take a routine you used to build strength and muscle and make it more conditioning based simply by dropping the weight and cramming in more rounds in less time. Like this one!*

Single-arm swing × **10 reps**
Turkish get up × **1 rep**
Switch sides and repeat.

Prescription: AMRAP 20 minutes.
Weight: Use a weight that is between your 5- and 8-rep TGU max.

The Old-School Lead-In

Back when I practiced bare-knuckle boxing, this was the warm-up or "lead-in" to every training session. I loved it then. I love it now.

Kettlebell swing	×	**30 seconds**
Plank	×	**60 seconds**
Skip rope or hop in place (active recovery)	×	**90 seconds**

Prescription: AMRAP 20 minutes.

Weight: Men use 20 to 28 kg; women, 8 to 20 kg.

Recycle!

Single-arm clean   × 1 rep
Single-arm squat   × 1 rep
Reverse lunge to overhead × 1 rep (use the momentum out of the
    press   lunge to assist with the press)
Repeat 5 times before setting the kettlebell down.
Switch sides and repeat.

Prescription: AMRAP 20 minutes.
Weight: Men use 16 to 20 kg; women, 8 to 12 kg.

The Potato

What's the story behind this workout name? No idea.

Single-arm swing   × 3 reps
Single-arm clean and press × 3 reps
Snatch   × 3 reps
Reverse Turkish get up   × 1 rep
Switch sides and repeat.

Prescription: AMRAP 20 minutes.
Weight: Men use 12 to 20 kg; women, 8 to 12 kg.

Trifecta

Note: *Here's a video of this workout, which demos the crush curl.*

Kettlebell swing × **1 rep**
Crush curl   × **1 rep**
Push-up   × **1 rep**
Continue for 30 seconds without resting, then rest 1 to 2 minutes.

Prescription: AMRAP 20 minutes.
Weight: Men use 16 to 20 kg; women, 8 to 12 kg.

1 Kettlebell + 220 Reps = You'll Thank Me Later

WORKOUT
8

Note: *Basic exercises, but lots of reps. You'll be performing a 10- to 1-rep ladder of several exercises. So, you'll
start by doing 10 reps of each exercise, then 9 reps of each, and so on. Good
luck! (Handily, I have a video of this routine as well.)*

Kettlebell swing	×	**10 reps**
Goblet squat	×	**10 reps**
Crush curl	×	**10 reps**
Push-up	×	**10 reps**

*Repeat, removing 1 rep of each exercise every round until you reach
1 rep.*

Prescription: Try to complete the entire workout, or as much as you
can, in 20 minutes.
Weight: Men use 16 to 24 kg; women, 8 to 16 kg.

Just Swings and Push-Ups

This used to be a standard finisher in my kettlebell boot-camp classes (which I taught for years). It's a foolproof way to crank the metabolism by performing frequent level changes (getting on and off the ground).

Kettlebell swing × 10 reps + push-up × 10 reps
Kettlebell swing × 10 reps + push-up × 9 reps
Repeat, removing 1 push-up rep every round until you reach
    kettlebell swing × 10 reps + push-up × 1 rep.

Prescription: AMRAP 20 minutes.
Weight: Men use 20 to 28 kg; women, 12 to 20 kg.

Just Swings and Squats

Kettlebell swing × 10 reps + goblet squat × 10 reps
Kettlebell swing × 10 reps + goblet squat × 9 reps
Repeat, removing 1 goblet squat rep every round until you reach
kettlebell swing × 10 reps + goblet squat × 1 rep.

Prescription: AMRAP 20 minutes.
Weight: Men use 16 to 28 kg; women, 8 to 16 kg.

Up We Go

Kettlebell swing   ×   1 rep
Goblet squat   ×   1 rep
Push-up   ×   1 rep
Repeat, adding 1 rep of each exercise every round. If technique fails,
start over with 1 rep of each exercise.

Prescription: AMRAP 20 minutes.
Weight: Men use 16 to 24 kg; women, 8 to 16 kg.

Staggered

Note: *The staggered 8, 5, 3, 2 rep sequence (no, I didn't forget 7, 6, or 4!) works extremely well for conditioning complexes. Just the right sort of intensity wave. Check it out.*

Single-arm snatch	×	**8 reps/side**
Single-arm squat	×	**5 reps/side**
Single-arm military press	×	**3 reps/side**
Single-arm row	×	**2 reps/side**

Prescription: AMRAP 20 minutes.
Weight: Men use 12 to 20 kg; women, 8 to 12 kg.

Single-Arm Swing Mountain

Climb as high as you can . . .

Single-arm swing × 1 rep/side + plank × 5 seconds
Single-arm swing × 2 reps/side + plank × 5 seconds
Single-arm swing × 3 reps/side + plank × 5 seconds
Repeat, adding 1 rep of the exercise every round. If technique fails,
    drop back to 1 rep and start over.

Prescription: Continue for 20 minutes.

Weight: Men use 12 to 20 kg; women, 8 to 12 kg.

Snatch Test!

The snatch test has been something of a rite of passage in the kettlebell world for, well, decades, at this point. The standard for this is to eventually hit 100 snatches in just 5 minutes with 24 kg for men, 16 kg for women. Either way, a truly phenomenal conditioning routine.

Snatch × 100 reps

Prescription: Complete all reps as quickly as possible (generally switching hands every 10 to 20 reps).

Weight: Men use 16 to 24 kg; women, 8 to 16 kg.

Contrast Swings!

Note: *This workout is particularly fun with an extremely wide weight contrast—that is, go very heavy for the start-stop swings and quite light for the two-hand swings. You can alternate between plank and hollow hold at each round, if you'd like.*

Line up one heavy and one light kettlebell for kettlebell swings and perform the following without rest:

At the heavy bell: start-stop swing   ×   **5 reps**
At the light bell: kettlebell swing   ×   **15 reps**
Plank or hollow hold   ×   **20 seconds**

Prescription: AMRAP 20 minutes.

Weight: For the heaviest bell, men use 28 to 32 kg; women, 16 to 24 kg.

Contrast Get Ups!

Note: *For the super slow Turkish get up, essentially, per-form as few reps as possible while moving the entire time; it should look slow motion! For the speedy Turkish get up, perform them as quickly as possible while maintaining good technique.*

Complete the following without rest:

Super slow Turkish get up × 2 minutes (switch sides every rep)
Speedy Turkish get up   × 2 minutes (switch sides every rep)
Kettlebell swing   × 10 reps
Rest and repeat.

Prescription: AMRAP 20 minutes. Complete the TGUs and swings without rest in between until you've completed a set.
Weight: Men use 16 to 20 kg; women, 8 to 12 kg.

Get Up!

Speedy Turkish get up: repeat until technical failure
(RIGHT)

Speedy Turkish get up: repeat until technical failure
(LEFT)

Single-arm kettlebell swing   ×   10 reps/side

Rest and repeat.

Prescription: AMRAP 20 minutes.

Weight: Men use 12 to 20 kg; women, 8 to 12 kg.

Construction Project

Note: *The goal of this workout is to see how large of a complex you can build by adding both exercises and reps as you move along. Use common sense, of course, and don't push beyond proper technique (but still push!).*

Double clean	×	1 rep
Push-up	×	1 rep
Double clean	×	1 rep
Front squat	×	1 rep
Push-up	×	1 rep
Double clean	×	1 rep
Front squat	×	1 rep
Double military press	×	1 rep
Push-up	×	1 rep

Repeat, adding 1 rep of each exercise every round. If technique fails, start over with 1 rep of each exercise.

Prescription: AMRAP 20 minutes.

Weight: Men use two 16- to 20-kg kettlebells; women, two 8- to 12-kg bells.

Crazy 8s

Single-arm swing	× 8 reps/side
Single-arm clean	× 8 reps/side
Snatch	× 8 reps/side
Single-arm military press	× 8 reps/side
Single-arm push press	× 8 reps/side
Single-arm squat	× 8 reps/side
Reverse lunge	× 8 reps/side
Kettlebell swing	× 8 reps

Prescription: AMRAP 20 minutes.

Weight: Men use 12 to 20 kg; women, 8 to 12 kg.

Quick 300!

Note: *This workout is a taster of my larger 300 Swings Kettlebell Challenge. If you like the painful simplicity of this routine, see appendix 1 for more.*

Kettlebell swing × 300 reps

> **Prescription:** Complete all reps, or as close to that many as possible, in 20 minutes or less. Break up the sets and reps however you want or need (if you want specific ideas, see appendix 1).
> **Weight:** Men use 12 to 24 kg; women, 8 to 16 kg.

Playing the Hits

Every minute on the minute:

Minute 1: Single-arm swing × 5 reps (RIGHT)
Minute 2: Turkish get up × 1 rep (RIGHT)
Minute 3: Single-arm swing × 5 reps (LEFT)
Minute 4: Turkish get up × 1 rep (LEFT)

> **Prescription:** AMRAP 20 minutes.
> **Weight:** Men use 12 to 20 kg; women, 8 to 16 kg.

The Viking

Note: *Fifteen seconds of work followed by 15 seconds of rest for some extended amount of time (10 minutes, 15 minutes, maybe even 30 minutes) is one of the surest ways to increase your ability to go the distance while learning to maintain poise under pressure. When it comes to kettlebells, two exercises work particularly well within this scheme because of their "not too fast, not too slow" rhythm: snatch and push press.*

Snatch × 15 seconds ON / 15 seconds OFF (work for 15 seconds; rest for 15 seconds)
Switch sides every set.

> **Prescription:** AMRAP 20 minutes, trying not to take any additional rest.
>
> **Weight:** Men use 12 to 16 kg; women, 8 to 12 kg.

The Other Viking

Single-arm push press × 15 seconds ON / 15 seconds OFF (work for 15 seconds; rest for 15 seconds)
Switch sides every set.

> **Prescription:** AMRAP 20 minutes, trying not to take any additional rest.
> **Weight:** Men use 12 to 16 kg; women, 8 to 12 kg.

Kettlebell Inferno!

WORKOUT
24

Note: *This routine is also something of a cult classic; video can be found here:*

Kettlebell swing	×	2 reps
Single-arm swing	×	2 reps/side
Snatch	×	2 reps/side
Thruster	×	2 reps/side
Single-arm row	×	2 reps/side
Push-up	×	2 reps

Repeat, adding 2 reps of each exercise until you reach 10 reps, then go back down.

Prescription: Complete as much of the prescribed workout as possible in 20 minutes.
Weight: Men use 12 to 20 kg; women, 8 to 16 kg.

Piggy

Kettlebell swing × 1 rep
Goblet squat   × 1 rep
Push-up   × 1 rep
Repeat, adding 1 rep of each exercise each set until you reach 4 reps,
*   then go back down.*

Prescription: AMRAP 20 minutes.
Weight: Men use 20 to 24 kg; women, 8 to 16 kg.

Tabata Swings!

Note: *Many of you will recognize the name Tabata, but for those who don't, this is a form of high-intensity interval training. It's seriously great, and works perfectly with kettlebell swings.*

Kettlebell swing   × **20 seconds**
Rest   × **10 seconds**
Repeat for 4 minutes.
Then, rest 2 minutes and start again.

Prescription: Repeat 3 times.
Weight: Men use 20 to 24 kg; women, 8 to 16 kg.

Tabata Snatches!

Single-arm swing   × **20 seconds**
Rest   × **10 seconds**
Repeat for 4 minutes.
Then, rest 2 minutes and start again.

Prescription: Repeat 3 times.
Weight: Men use 16 to 20 kg; women 6 to 12 kg.

Big Hero 6

I thought the movie of the same title was good—not great, but good. Thanks for coming to my review.

Single-arm swing	×	6 reps
Single-arm clean	×	6 reps
Single-arm press	×	6 reps
Single-arm snatch	×	6 reps
Single-arm squat	×	6 reps
Reverse lunge	×	6 reps

Switch sides and repeat.

Prescription: AMRAP 20 minutes.
Weight: Men use 16 to 20 kg; women, 6 to 12 kg.

Bigger Hero 6

Double swing × 6 reps
Double clean × 6 reps
Double press × 6 reps
Double clean × 6 reps
Front squat   × 6 reps
Double row   × 6 reps

Prescription: AMRAP 20 minutes.

Weight: Men use two 16- to 20-kg kettlebells; women, two 6- to 12-kg bells.

2 of Everything

Single-arm swing   × 2 reps/side
Single-arm clean and press   × 2 reps/side
Single-arm snatch   × 2 reps/side
Turkish get up   × 2 reps/side

Prescription: AMRAP 20 minutes.

Weight: Men use 12 to 20 kg; women, 6 to 12 kg.

MOBILITY WORKOUTS

Note: *With mobility workouts, we're far less concerned about hitting a particular intensity as we are when trying to gain strength and muscle. For this reason, I am simply going to prescribe general weight ranges that work well for most people when performing these routines, but feel free to adjust accordingly, and when it doubt, err on the side of going lighter rather than heavier with these. We're really after maximally confident control (as opposed to maximal muscle punishment) through range of motion with these workouts, so you can feel limbered and restored.*

Jelly Roll

WORKOUT
1

This routine is, like so many others, super simple, but don't underestimate it. The combination of get ups, glute bridges, and plank works honest wonders for the hips and shoulders. **Note:** *If you need a refresher on the hip bridge, these are the steps: Lie on your back, squeeze your glutes, drive your hips up, and hold.*

Turkish get up	×	**1 rep (RIGHT)**
Hip bridge	×	**30 seconds**
Turkish get up	×	**1 rep (LEFT)**
Plank	×	**30 seconds**

Prescription: Repeat 4 times. Finish with 50 body-weight squats, if time permits.
Weight: Men use 12 to 20 kg; women, 8 to 12 kg.

Slow Down

Note: *Little tip for the single-leg deadlift, which is featured in this routine: Hold the kettlebell in the opposite arm of your planted leg. In other words, if your right leg is working, hold the kettlebell with your left arm. Also, if you need a little balance help starting out, just use your nonworking arm to place a finger or two on something for support, like a table or railing.*

Single-leg deadlift	×	10 reps/side
Single-arm swing	×	10 reps/side
Windmill	×	5 reps/side
Super slow Turkish get up	×	2 reps/side

Prescription: AMRAP 15 to 20 minutes.

Weight: Men use 12 to 16 kg; women, 8 to 12 kg.

Unwind a Little

Note: *For this routine, you'll perform a snatch, hold the kettlebell at the top, then get into position to perform a windmill, finish the windmill, and then snatch the kettlebell back down, and repeat. It's an awesome flow that stretches out just about everything while providing a pretty powerful cardio hit as well.*

Snatch to windmill × **5 reps/side**
Goblet squat   × **5 reps**

Prescription: AMRAP 15 minutes.
Weight: Men use 12 to 16 kg; women, 8 to 12 kg.

Breather

Note: *This routine features breathing get ups. What are breathing get ups, you ask? Simply this:* Take one full and deep breath at each stage of the TGU. *This forces you to slow down and really nail each segment of the exercise. Moreover, breath control while exercising is an important skill in its own right, and this is an effective way to practice that. Enjoy!*

Breathing Turkish get up × 1 rep/side

Prescription: AMRAP 15 to 20 minutes, trying to move continuously.
Weight: Men use 12 to 16 kg; women, 6 to 8 kg.

Stretchy Pants

Everybody loves a good pair of stretchy pants, no?

Snatch	×	10 reps (RIGHT)
Clean and push press	×	5 reps (RIGHT)
Snatch	×	10 reps (LEFT)
Clean and push press	×	5 reps (LEFT)

Prescription: AMRAP 15 to 20 minutes.

Weight: Use a light weight for this workout: Men, 12 to 16 kg; women, 6 to 12 kg.

Breathing Ladder v.1

Note: *As the name implies, intentional breathing is a big part of this routine. Consider this a form of breath practice, where you try to inhale for 4 seconds, exhale for 6 to 8 seconds. You'll be performing a 1- to 10-rep kettlebell swing ladder. After every set of swings, take as many long, slow, deep breaths as swings performed.*

Kettlebell swing × 1 rep + deep breath × 1 rep
Kettlebell swing × 2 reps + deep breath × 2 reps
Repeat, adding 1 rep of the exercise and deep breath until you reach
    10 reps and breaths. Go back down the ladder from 10 reps to
    1 rep if desired.

Prescription: AMRAP 20 minutes.
Weight: Men use 16 to 20 kg; women, 8 to 12 kg.

Breathing Ladder v.2

Note: *You'll be performing a 1- to 10-rep goblet squat ladder. After every set of squats, take as many long, slow, deep breaths as squats performed.*

Goblet squat × 1 rep + deep breath × 1 rep
Goblet squat × 2 reps + deep breath × 2 reps
Repeat, adding 1 rep of the exercise and deep breath until you reach
10 reps and breaths. Go back down the ladder from 10 reps to
1 rep if desired.

Prescription: AMRAP 20 minutes.
Weight: Men use 12 to 20 kg; women, 6 to 12 kg.

Hunky Dory

Single-arm swing	× **30 seconds/side**
Clean	× **30 seconds/side**
Push press	× **30 seconds/side**
Windmill	× **30 seconds/side**
Kettlebell halo	× **30 seconds/side**
Hindu push-up	× **30 seconds**
Plank	× **30 seconds**

Prescription: Repeat for 3 rounds (or as much as you can get done in 20 minutes).

Weight: Men use 12 to 20 kg; women, 6 to 12 kg.

Sidewinder

Note: *This routine is stellar for shoulder mobility and stability and getting strong at weird angles. However, there is
a lot of overhead work here, so if necessary, place the kettlebell down for
extra rest if things begin to feel a bit too wobbly.*

Snatch	×	10 reps/side
Windmill	×	2 reps/side
Turkish get up	×	1 rep/side
Snatch	×	8 reps/side
Windmill	×	2 reps/side
Turkish get up	×	1 rep/side
Snatch	×	6 reps/side
Windmill	×	2 reps/side
Turkish get up	×	1 rep/side
Snatch	×	4 reps/side
Windmill	×	2 reps/side
Turkish get up	×	1 rep/side
Snatch	×	2 reps/side
Windmill	×	2 reps/side
Turkish get up	×	1 rep/side

Prescription: AMRAP 20 minutes.
Weight: Men use 12 to 16 kg; women, 6 to 8 kg.

The Contortionist

For those of you who need to fit into awkward places . . .

Hip bridge   ×   **20 seconds**
Plank   ×   **20 seconds**
Do 3 rounds. Then . . .
**Turkish get up to windmill (perform 1 windmill at the top of the get
    up) × 1 rep/side**

Prescription: AMRAP 15 minutes.
Weight: Men use 8 to 16 kg; women, 6 to 12 kg.

Extend

Kettlebell swing   ×   **15 reps**
Hip bridge   ×   **20 seconds**
Single-leg deadlift   ×   **8 reps/side**
Turkish get up   ×   **1 rep/side**

Prescription: AMRAP 15 to 20 minutes.
Weight: Men use 12 to 20 kg; women, 6 to 12 kg.

Like Bamboo

A workout to make you strong and flexible, like bamboo!

Windmill   × **8 reps (RIGHT)**
Single-leg deadlift   × **8 reps (RIGHT)**
Hindu push-up   × **8 reps**
Switch sides and repeat.

Prescription: AMRAP 15 to 20 minutes.
Weight: Men use 12 to 20 kg; women, 6 to 12 kg.

In 4 Repairs

March in place or skip rope	×	20 seconds
Kettlebell swing	×	15 reps
Goblet squat	×	10 reps
Push-up	×	5 reps

Prescription: AMRAP 20 minutes.

Weight: Men use 12 to 20 kg; women, 8 to 12 kg.

Light and Easy

Goblet squat	×	5 reps
Clean and push press	×	5 reps/side
Windmill	×	5 reps/side
Kettlebell halo	×	5 reps/side
Goblet squat	×	5 reps

Prescription: AMRAP 15 minutes.

Weight: Men use 16 kg; women, 8 kg.

Slow Then Fast

Note: *When performing super slow get ups, try to make
each rep at least 30 seconds. Super speedy get ups should
be performed as quickly as possible without distorting technique.*

Super slow Turkish get up	×	2 reps/side
Super speedy Turkish get up	×	2 reps/side

Prescription: Alternate between going slow and fast through the TGU
(always maintaining good form!) for 15 to 20 minutes.
Weight: Men use 12 to 16 kg; women, 6 to 8 kg.

Something for the Abs

Note: *The hollow hold to plank combo is perhaps my favorite "love to hate" direct core strengthener. Just remember to keep your abs braced and rib cage tucked when performing the hollow holds—don't arch your back!*

Kettlebell swing	×	15 reps
Hollow hold	×	20 seconds
Plank	×	20 seconds

Prescription: Do 5 rounds.

Weight: Men use 12 to 16 kg; women, 8 to 12 kg.

CONCLUSION

In all matters of life, we ought to seek efficiency and effectiveness. To do things right and to do the right things. This is the heart of minimalism: not wasting efforts and not cluttering our lives with fluff, filler, and BS. To take a machete to the weeds that clog the path to our goals.

I hope as we near the end of this book, you can see, obviously and most assuredly, how minimalism can be that machete, slashing the excess that keeps fitness programs bloated and fitness enthusiasts from reaching their goals with alacrity and vim. How minimalism in fitness is the anti-dote to the marketing claptrap that prevails in much of the industry, luring well-meaning folks into a wasteland of ineffective—and, frankly, weird—exercises and years of minimal returns.

From the kettlebell swing to the Turkish get up, each exercise chosen for this microtome has been selected for its efficiency and effectiveness. Each one simply *is* the right tool for the job, specifically when the job is to become good to great at many different skills, never fretting about being the best in the world at a particular one but rather becoming impressive across the board (who wouldn't want *that*?). This is what it means to become an expert-generalist. And as we've seen throughout these pages, minimalism is the perfect bedrock on which to build the foundation for generalism.

When we align our goals to a generalist perspective, great things can happen. We can avoid injury and burnout. We can blast through plateaus that have dogged us for far too long. We can be the envy of our annual neighborhood grill out, and we can haul a ton of mulch around the yard without feeling broken and defeated when the last chip falls.

Generalism is freeing. When we apply a minimalist fitness philosophy to our goal of generalism, we find that we have the time, energy, and capabilities to get the work done. And by training to the goal of a great many skills, we are free to be excellent. To see a pull-up bar and blast out reps. To see an obstacle—a heavy piano, a mile run, etc.—and overcome it. And to never be intimidated again when somebody declares the floor is lava. In short, to find ourselves in situations where our confidence once wavered but now we are unflappable. These are no small things, and our ability to do these things can affect all aspects of our lives. Train toward generalism using minimalism and be encouraged, capable, strong, and harder to kill.

The heart of any fitness book, quite naturally, is its content—the training plan, the eating regimen, etc.—coupled with the inspiration to put that content to consistent use. A coach, properly understood, isn't just some abstract navigation aide but an active trail guide and personally interested party; ideally, they are the spark that ignites your enthusiasm and keeps you engaged and energetic, especially when moving through tough terrain and sticky plateaus.

As your coach, I want you to try this mental exercise: Envision yourself a decade from now. Unless you're already celebrating your centennial (and if so, hats off for picking up my book; in fact, let me buy you a beer—ten years from now), you'll likely be anticipating at least another ten years. Ten years is a lot of time, certainly enough time to make serious and dramatic changes. That time will pass, regardless. The real question is, how will you use it?

Here's my suggestion: If you're planning to stick around for another year, five years, or even half a century, why not make the most of it? Why not shift away from quick fixes and focus on the exhilaration—imagined now, but entirely possible later—of looking back and seeing the absolute specimen you've become.

Why? Because the usual notion that if people fail to reach their fitness goals, it's because they didn't want them badly enough is, in my opinion, false. I believe people genuinely desire and care about their fitness goals. The challenge is balancing these goals with other aspects of life—comfort, friendships, social acceptance—which often take precedence. These aren't negative in themselves, but they can conflict with our fitness aspirations, for sure. Adopting a long-term view, imagining the future self you could develop through consistent, minimalist, and effective practice, can profoundly shift your mindset. Compare yourself in ten years with and without this commitment. How does each vision make you feel? What actions are you inspired to take?

This perspective has been a hugely propulsive force in driving me to make tough choices and put in the daily effort that (like many) I'd rather cast aside for video games and easy carbs. Of course, I've never been perfect; I stumble like anyone, early and often. But here's the thing about that: You don't need to be perfect; in fact, striving for perfection is sometimes the enemy of progress because of the impossible expectation you set for yourself. Just strive to work with full trust in the process.

At this point, I'm tempted to finish with the cliché "Let's get started," but honestly, we're already on our path, making such a beginning redundant. Our task is to keep the pace and press ahead. Strong ON!

APPENDIX 1
The 300 Swings Kettlebell Challenge

I created the 300 Swings Kettlebell Challenge for people wanting a serious but single-minded fitness challenge. Something that efficiently torches calories, builds full-body functional strength, and conditions you like nothing else—all done with just one simple, fundamental exercise: the kettlebell swing.

The name of the challenge implies its objective: 300 kettlebell swings, done every day, for thirty days. That's right. Just remember, this is a challenge; it's supposed to be tough. Nevertheless, the Strong ON! motto applies even here: challenged, but successful.

The purpose of 300 swings? To provide you with a thirty-day relentless assault on unwanted body fat (and general bodily weakness) through the power of a kettlebell exercise many have grown to love to hate because of its ruthless efficiency. The high volume of swings allows you to really concentrate on sculpting the posterior chain, working those hamstrings, glutes, and lower-back muscles. Bonus result? What many affectionately refer to as "kettle-booty"—a set of buttocks that means business.

There are, of course, many other benefits of the 300 Swings challenge. Each session not only burns close to the calorie equivalent of uphill cross-country skiing but also comes with the added bonus of involving no uphill cross-country skiing whatsoever. Your conditioning, too, will quickly become unsurpassed, as many of these routines will push you right to the limit of what you're currently capable of, expanding your capability over time. Moreover, the 300 Swings challenge is truly an opportunity to master kettlebell swing technique. Embrace the spirit of Bruce Lee, and instead of thinking of it as 300 swings, focus on one swing repeated 300 times—perfect technique with every rep. Your final swing should look just like, or at least very close to, your first swing in every workout.

How to achieve this? First, set the intention. Approach training as a form of movement practice, with your mind set on mastering technique through purposeful repetition, constantly reminding yourself of the elements of a proper kettlebell swing (flat back, hips back, etc.). Second, if necessary, make commonsense adjustments, either to weight or reps or whatever you need to ensure proper technique is never sacrificed for the sole sake of getting one's reps in.

Now, let's address the elephant in the room—300 swings is a substantial number. I get that. But here's the exciting part: Not every workout is the same, even if the ultimate objective of the workout is. In other words, we don't stick to a single weight, nor do we perform identical sets and reps day in and day out. Our approach is diverse and adaptable. At times, we swing heavy; at other times, we go lighter. We also play with timing; some days, we aim to complete all 300 reps in short bursts, while other days, we spread the reps throughout the day, enjoying metabolic boosts before each meal, while allowing for more recovery.

Given the high frequency of training, we get creative in manipulating various workout variables, like intensity and density, to ensure we train hard without overdoing it. Thus, it's paramount that you follow the provided workouts meticulously during the 300 Swings challenge. This structured approach ensures you make the most of your effort and maximize the benefits of this, indeed, quite challenging challenge.

Final words of advice before we look at the program: If this is your first time running the 300 Swings challenge, I recommend running it alone—that is, without combining it with another program, including those in this book. If, on the other hand, you're a 300 Swings veteran, then you can combine 300 Swings with another program, including those in this book, but here's my advice for that: Break up the routines. Don't perform them back-to-back if you can help it. Rather, perform your 300 swings in the morning and then your other workout routine at lunch or after work. Or the other way around. (Generally, I recommend doing the more difficult workout first.)

As for how often to run the 300 Swings challenge, my general advice is just once or twice per year. Four would be the max; any more than that and I think you not only risk overdoing it but also begin to miss out on the benefits provided from other training plans, particularly those featured in this book. From my experience (having now led tens of thousands of people through this protocol), 300 Swings is the perfect New Year's fitness endeavor. I know that can be a little cliché, but there really is something about starting the new year off with an exciting, community-based fitness romp. Indeed, the Strong ON! community typically does launch into 300 Swings every New Year's, and I cannot emphasize how powerful community support is when running a fitness challenge. If you haven't already, I strongly encourage you to join our free Strong ON! social media community.

Okay, sorry for prattling on. I think I got the bare essentials out. Time now to actually look at what the 300 Swings challenge consists of. But wait: If this is your first time running 300 Swings, we also have a beginner ramp-up protocol, which I recommend using before you being the full thirty-day challenge. See toward the end of the appendix for that.

THE 300 SWINGS 30-DAY KETTLEBELL CHALLENGE

Here are the workouts to be performed in order for the next thirty days of our 300 Swings Kettlebell Challenge. Before we dive in, it's important to note that specific recommendations are provided for some routines, but these are just general guidelines. You should adjust the weight based on your current strength, conditioning, and size.

Additionally, some routines suggest using either a heavy or light weight, leaving it to your discretion to determine what qualifies as heavy or light for you in relation to the workout prescribed. When opting for a heavier weight, challenge yourself, of course, but always ensure you can maintain impeccable technique throughout the workout.

Common sense should guide you throughout this challenge. If you find that you need extra rest, especially because of deteriorating technique, take it. If you're experiencing excessive soreness or fatigue, it's perfectly acceptable to shorten a set or two—or even an entire workout. The purpose of a worthwhile fitness challenge is to push your limits, encouraging them to expand—not to exceed those limits to the point of potential injury or burnout.

THE 300 SWINGS RAMP-UP PROGRAM

Looking to ease your way into the 300 Swings Kettlebell Challenge? Try my weeklong ramp-up program. The aim here is to gradually increase your kettlebell swing volume before fully diving into the full 300-rep challenge. Use a weight that provides a comfortable challenge for the prescribed reps, and feel free to arrange the sets and reps in any way you prefer (sets of 10, 5, 15, etc.).

- **Day 1:** 100 swings
- **Day 2:** 50 swings
- **Day 3:** 50 swings
- **Day 4:** 100 swings
- **Day 5:** 150 swings
- **Day 6:** 250 swings
- **Day 7:** 50 swings

Remember, you know your body best. Challenge it when it tries to quit prematurely, but also listen attentively to the signals it gives you. Often, it's better to respect your body's current limits and live to swing another day.

Ready to get started?

Day 1

Kettlebell swing × 30 reps

Perform 10 times.

Weight: Men use 12 to 20 kg; women, 8 to 12 kg.

Day 2

Set 40 minutes on the clock.

Perform a set of swings at the top of every minute, completing 300 swings *before* the 40 minutes expire.

Weight: Men use 16 to 24 kg; women, 8 to 16 kg.

Day 3

Heavy start-stop swings × 10 reps (park the kettlebell between every rep)

Light single-arm swings × 10 reps/side

Complete 10 total sets.

Day 4

Free day: Kettlebell swing × 300 reps, however you want with whatever weight you want. (Consider lighter swings if you're sore.)

Day 5

At the top of every minute, perform:

> *Minute 1:* Kettlebell swing × 5 reps
>
> *Minute 2:* Kettlebell swing × 5 reps
>
> *Minute 3:* Kettlebell swing × 10 reps
>
> *Minute 4:* Kettlebell swing × 10 reps
>
> *Minute 5:* Kettlebell swing × 20 reps
>
> *Minute 6:* Kettlebell swing × 20 reps
>
> *Minute 7:* Kettlebell swing × 30 reps
>
> *Complete 3 times.*
>
> *Weight:* Men use 16 to 24 kg; women, 8 to 16 kg.

Day 6

> *Free day:* Kettlebell swing × 300 reps, however you want with whatever weight you want. (Consider lighter swings if you're sore.)

Day 7

> Kettlebell swing × 300 reps . . . in as *few* sets as possible.
>
> *Weight:* Men use 16 to 24 kg; women, 8 to 16 kg.

Day 8

> Kettlebell swing × 10 reps
>
> *Perform 30 times.*
>
> *Weight:* Men use 20 to 28 kg; women, 12 to 20 kg.

Day 9

Kettlebell swing × 30 reps

Perform 10 times.

Weight: Men use 16 to 20 kg; women, 8 to 12 kg.

Day 10

Free day: Kettlebell swing × 300 reps, however you want with whatever weight you want. (Consider lighter swings if you're sore.)

Day 11

At the top of every minute, perform:

Minute 1: Kettlebell swing × 30 reps

Minute 2: Kettlebell swing × 5 reps

Minute 3: Kettlebell swing × 5 reps

Minute 4: Kettlebell swing × 5 reps

Minute 5: Kettlebell swing × 5 reps

Complete 6 times.

Weight: Men use 16 to 24 kg; women, 8 to 16 kg.

Day 12

Kettlebell swing × 300 reps, as *quickly* as possible.

Weight: Men use 16 to 20 kg; women, 8 to 12 kg.

Day 13

Kettlebell swing × 300 reps, in as *few* sets as possible.

Weight: Men use 20 to 24 kg; women, 12 to 16 kg.

Day 14

Free day: Kettlebell swing × 300 reps, however you want with whatever weight you want. (Consider lighter swings if you're sore.)

Day 15

Free day: Kettlebell swing × 300 reps, however you want with whatever weight you want. (Consider lighter swings if you're sore.)

Day 16

Kettlebell swing × 5 reps

Kettlebell swing × 10 reps

Kettlebell swing × 15 reps

Kettlebell swing × 20 reps

Perform 6 times.

Weight: Men use 24 kg; women, 16 kg.

Day 17

Single-arm kettlebell swing × 150 reps/side, as quickly as possible.

Weight: Men use 16 kg; women, 8 kg.

Day 18

Perform as many good, *crisp* swings as you can in a single set.

Subtract 5 reps and perform *that many reps* per set until 300 swings are complete (e.g., if you get 20 reps your first set, then the rest of your sets should be 15 reps).

Weight: Men use 24 kg; women, 16 kg.

Day 19

Free day: Kettlebell swing × 300 reps, however you want with whatever weight you want. (Consider lighter swings if you're sore.)

Day 20

At the top of every minute, perform:

Minute 1: Kettlebell swing × 30 reps

Minute 2: Kettlebell swing × 5 reps

Minute 3: Kettlebell swing × 5 reps

Minute 4: Kettlebell swing × 5 reps

Minute 5: Kettlebell swing × 5 reps

Complete 6 times.

Weight: Men use 16 to 24 kg; women, 8 to 16 kg.

Day 21

Heavy start-stop swings × 10 reps (park the kettlebell between every rep)

Light single-arm swings × 10 reps/side

Complete 10 total sets.

Day 22

Perform a 2- to 10-rep ladder, going up by twos (a set of 2 swings, 4 swings . . . up to 10 swings, then go back down, repeating 10 swings).

Complete 5 times through.

Weight: Men use 24 kg; women, 16 kg.

Day 23

Free day: Kettlebell swing × 300 reps, however you want with whatever weight you want. (Consider lighter swings if you're sore.)

Day 24

Single-arm swings × 75 reps/side, as quickly as possible

Hand-to-hand swings × 150 reps

Weight: Men use 16 kg; women, 8 kg.

Day 25

Kettlebell swing × 300 reps, in as *few* sets as possible.

Weight: Men use 16 to 20 kg; women, 8 to 12 kg.

Day 26

At the top of every minute, perform:

> *Minute 1:* Kettlebell swing × 20 reps
>
> *Minute 2:* Kettlebell swing × 5 reps
>
> *Minute 3:* Kettlebell swing × 10 reps
>
> *Minute 4:* Kettlebell swing × 5 reps
>
> *Minute 5:* Kettlebell swing × 20 reps
>
> *Complete 5 times.*
>
> *Weight:* Men use 16 to 24 kg; women, 8 to 16 kg.

Day 27

> *Free day:* Kettlebell swing × 300 reps, however you want with whatever weight you want. (Consider lighter swings if you're sore.)

Day 28

> *Heavy* start-stop swing × 5 reps (park the kettlebell between every rep)
>
> *Light* kettlebell swing × 10 reps
>
> *Complete 20 total sets.*

Day 29

> Single-arm swing × 10 reps (RIGHT)—*complete 10 times*
>
> Single-arm swing × 10 reps (LEFT)—*complete 10 times*
>
> Kettlebell swing × 100 reps, in as *few* sets as possible
>
> *Weight:* Men use 16 to 20 kg; women, 8 to 12 kg.

Day 30

Kettlebell swing × 300 reps, with crisp, flawless technique as quickly as possible.

The goal is to complete all reps in 15 minutes or less.

Weight: Men use 24 kg; women, 16 kg.

Bonus 1

Kettlebell swing × 10 reps

Kettlebell swing × 15 reps

Kettlebell swing × 15 reps

Kettlebell swing × 30 reps

Kettlebell swing × 30 reps

Perform 3 times through.

Weight: Men use 16 to 24 kg; women, 8 to 16 kg.

Bonus 2

At the top of every minute, perform:

Minute 1: Kettlebell swing × 20 reps

Minute 2: Kettlebell swing × 5 reps

Minute 3: Kettlebell swing × 5 reps

Minute 4: Kettlebell swing × 5 reps

Minute 5: Kettlebell swing × 25 reps

Complete 5 times.

Weight: Men use 16 to 24 kg; women, 8 to 16 kg.

Bonus 3

Set 30 minutes on the clock.

Perform a set of swings of however many reps you want at the top of every minute.

Complete 300 swings *before* the 30 minutes expire.

Weight: Men use 16 to 24 kg; women, 8 to 16 kg.

APPENDIX 2

The World's Simplest Scientific Eating Plan

We don't need to emphasize the importance of nutrition; it's clear that what you eat significantly impacts your progress, whether you're striving to lose weight or gain muscle. What may not be as evident is precisely how to eat to achieve your specific goals. That's what we aim to clarify here.

The purpose of this brief appendix is to distill the essentials of intelligent eating—proposing a nutritional approach that's both scientifically sound and adaptable to individual preferences.

Let's get right to it.

CALORIES AND PROTEIN INTAKE: THE CORNERSTONES

Effective nutrition boils down to two fundamental factors: calorie and protein intake. If your goal is to lose weight, you'll generally need to decrease calorie consumption. Conversely, if you want to gain weight, you should increase your caloric intake. In both cases, elevating protein intake (assuming you aren't eating at such levels already) can significantly benefit you. How so? Well, while it's often thought that various diets result in comparable fat loss when calorie intake is equal, several studies suggest a distinct advantage for high-protein diets.[5] As researcher Layne Norton points out, "The results of these experiments show quite clearly that high protein diets have a metabolic fat loss advantage compared to normal/low protein diets. What's more, a high protein diet has been shown to be superior to normal/low protein diets in maintaining muscle mass and improving body composition during a diet."[6] This highlights protein's pivotal role in effective fat loss and muscle preservation.

UNDERSTANDING ENERGY BALANCE

Weight loss and weight gain ultimately come down to energy balance. If you consume more energy (calories) than you expend, your body stores the excess energy as fat, muscle, or both. Conversely, when you expend more energy than you consume, your body begins burning fat and, in some cases, muscle. To achieve your desired outcome—presumably, gaining muscle but not fat, or losing fat but not muscle—precision and regular intense exercise are key.

In short, the best way to preserve muscle while losing fat is to consume more protein and engage in resistance training. For those aiming to gain muscle rather than fat, lifting weights is essential, but it's crucial not to go overboard with calorie surplus to avoid excessive fat gain. What's overboard? Generally, a three hundred to five hundred daily calorie surplus is a safe lean-gains range. So, try to stay within that.

What Are Calories, Exactly?

Calories are a unit of measurement used to quantify the energy food provides when metabolized by the body. The three primary macronutrients contributing to calorie intake are carbohydrates, protein, and fat. While carbohydrates and protein provide roughly four calories per gram, fat is more calorically dense, providing around nine calories per gram.

PRACTICAL GUIDELINES FOR FAT LOSS AND MUSCLE GAIN

For Fat Loss

Reduce your daily calorie intake by 10 to 20 percent for five consecutive days.

Follow this with two consecutive days of caloric maintenance (which is the amount you need to maintain your current body weight). The standard approach for this would be a weekday/weekend split.

This cycling approach offers numerous benefits, including preserving lean muscle mass and preventing metabolic slowdown. It also provides nice (if not necessary) psychological relief.

To determine your caloric maintenance, consider using websites like caloriecalculator.net/calorie. Alternatively, for those who can't stand giving any more time to the internet, calculate your caloric maintenance simply by multiplying your weight in pounds by 16. For instance, if you weigh 150 pounds, your daily maintenance would be 150 × 16, which comes out to 2,400 calories. (Note: If you're highly active, use a multiplier of 18; for low activity levels, opt for 14.)

REALISTIC BODY FAT RANGES

Typically, most men can maintain a healthy body fat percentage between 10 to 20 percent, while women fall within the 18 to 28 percent range. Keep in mind that genetics and lifestyle factors affect your comfort level within these ranges, meaning some people will find the lower end of these ranges more difficult than others. Either way, striving to go below these ranges not only is increasingly difficult but also can lead to various health concerns (such as hormone imbalances, decreased immune function, and muscle loss) and result in lethargy and reduced libido. It's essential to set a realistic, sustainable target, somewhere within the ranges above.

For Muscle Gain

Increase calorie intake by 5 to 25 percent above maintenance calories daily.

For faster results and muscle gain, aim for the higher end; for more controlled fat levels, opt for the lower end.

Again, you can calculate your numbers using caloriecalculator.net /calorie or just use the method on page 193.

Additional Guidelines

1. Aim for at least one gram of protein per pound of your desired body weight daily.
2. Set fat intake between 20 and 35 percent of your daily calorie target and balance the rest with carbohydrates.
3. Consider tools like intermittent fasting or high-quality protein shakes to make calorie deficits more manageable. (Try replacing occasional meals with protein shakes, a strategy known to curb hunger and help meet protein targets.)
4. Additionally, consider supplementing with protein shakes in addition to meals when necessary.
5. While not obligatory, supplements like protein, caffeine (primarily on intense training days), and creatine can complement your nutrition plan, but they should never replace the fundamentals of a well-rounded training and nutrition regimen.
6. Take diet breaks. Generally speaking, when it comes to dieting for fat loss, you want to take a one- to two-week diet break (come back to caloric maintenance) every eight to twelve weeks. Doing so helps your results settle in while preventing metabolic downshifting and hormone imbalances. Cyclicality in dieting, as with training, is key.
7. Limit or eliminate hyperpalatable foods, such as those high in salt, sugar, and unhealthy fats, often associated with the slogan "You can't eat just one." Likewise, reduce or eliminate alcohol consumption. Success in fitness and nutrition often requires compromises;

you can't always have everything you want in your diet or lifestyle, so consider the trade-offs and choose accordingly. In other words, be an adult.

8. Prioritize sleep, aiming for at least seven to nine hours in a cool, dark room, as it significantly impacts both fat loss and muscle maintenance or growth. (This may seem outside the realm of eating, and in a sense it is, but it is flatly undeniable that sleep is the X factor that either facilitates or frustrates progress, other things equal. In other words, for many people, fixing their diet is tightly tied to fixing their sleep. So, this cannot be overlooked.)

This minimalist yet mostly comprehensive set of guidelines provides a straightforward, scientifically backed approach to nutrition. Follow whatever guidelines make the most sense for your goals—whether you want to emphasize fat loss or muscle gain—while understanding, especially if you're relatively new to exercise, that you can realistically recompose, or lose fat and gain muscle, at the same time. And be sure to take occasional diet breaks, where you just come back and rest at maintenance for a while, especially if pursuing fat loss.

ELEVATE YOUR KETTLEBELL GAME
Dive into These (Free) Resources

Ready to push your kettlebell skills to new heights? Dive into my renowned I Bet You Can't Do This Workout challenges. The best part? They're *free*.

Download fifteen masterfully curated kettlebell workout challenges, each designed to optimize muscle growth, fat loss, or endurance. Check them out.

Muscle: www.ChroniclesofStrength.com/KettlebellComplexesFor Muscle

Fat Loss: www.ChroniclesofStrength.com/KettlebellComplexesFor FatLoss

Endurance: www.ChroniclesofStrength.com/KettlebellComplexesFor Endurance

KETTLEBELL QUICKIES YOUTUBE CHANNEL

Subscribe to my Kettlebell Quickies YouTube channel for weekly "take you by the hand" time-efficient kettlebell workouts.

BEFORE YOU GO: WANT 101 MORE FREE KETTLEBELL WORKOUTS?!

That's right—I have rolled out an *additional* stash of 101 kettlebell workouts, and I'm sharing it for free. Pair these with the workouts from this book, and you're on track to an effectively diverse lifetime kettlebell regimen. Don't miss this fat-blasting, muscle-boosting treasure trove.

Grab your copy at www.101KettlebellWorkouts.com.

NOTES

1. Michael Fröhlich, Eike Emrich, and Dietmar Schmidtbleicher, "Outcome Effects of Single-Set Versus Multiple-Set Training—An Advanced Replication Study," *Research in Sports Medicine* 18, no. 3 (July 2010): 157–175, https://doi.org/10.1080/15438620903321045; Grant W. Ralston et al., "The Effect of Weekly Set Volume on Strength Gain: A Meta-analysis," *Sports Medicine* 47, no. 12 (December 2017): 2585–2601, https://doi.org/10.1007/s40279-017-0762-7.

2. Haruki Momma et al., "Muscle-Strengthening Activities Are Associated with Lower Risk and Mortality in Major Non-communicable Diseases: A Systematic Review and Meta-analysis of Cohort Studies," *British Journal of Sports Medicine* 56, no. 13 (July 2022): 755–763, https://doi.org/10.1136/bjsports-2021-105061.

3. Brad J. Schoenfeld, Dan Ogborn, and James W. Krieger, "Dose-Response Relationship Between Weekly Resistance Training Volume and Increases in Muscle Mass: A Systematic Review and Meta-analysis," *Journal of Sports Sciences* 35, no. 11 (July 2016): 1073–1082, https://doi.org/10.1080/02640414.2016.1210197. For a helpful overview of this research, see Jeff Nippard, "How to Train Like a Minimalist (More Gains in Less Time)," YouTube video, posted October 16, 2022, https://www.youtube.com/watch?v=xc4OtzAnVMI.

4. Jason P. Lake and Mike A. Lauder, "Kettlebell Swing Training Improves Maximal and Explosive Strength," *Journal of Strength and Conditioning Research* 26, no. 8 (August 2012): 2228–2233.

5. Bonnie J. Brehm et al., "A Randomized Trial Comparing a Very Low Carbohydrate Diet and a Calorie-Restricted Low Fat Diet on Body Weight and Cardiovascular Risk Factors in Healthy Women," *Journal of Clinical Endocrinology & Metabolism* 88, no. 4 (April 2003): 1617–1623; Donald K. Layman et al., "Dietary Protein and Exercise Have Additive Effects on Body Composition During Weight Loss in Adult Women," *Journal of Nutrition* 135, no. 8 (August 2005): 1903–1910.

6. Layne Norton. "Protein: More Than Just Muscle Building Substrate," *Biolayne*, May 1, 2016. https://biolayne.com/articles/nutrition/protein -just-muscle-building-substrate.

ABOUT THE AUTHOR

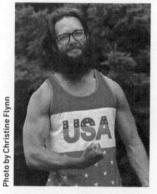

Photo by Christine Flynn

Writer, fitness coach, philosopher, guitarist, podcaster, tae kwon do black belt, entrepreneur, and devoted husband and father, **Pat Flynn** is a true expert-generalist. He propounds his belief in generalism—championing the mastery of diverse skills and epitomizing the spirit of a modern-day Renaissance man.

In fitness, he's trained everyone from Olympic athletes and Special Forces to thousands of regular folks looking to get in amazing shape in the least amount of time.

In testimony of his eclectic interests, Pat has published several books, including *How to Be Better at (Almost) Everything*, *The Best Argument for God*, and a collection of For Dummies kettlebell books, as well as hundreds of academic and popular-level articles about fitness, faith, and philosophy. He shares much of this generalist life philosophy on his two podcasts, *The Pat Flynn Show* and *Philosophy for the People*.

When not writing, training, and podcasting, Pat shares guitar licks on YouTube and gigs with a local band, playing '80s party metal tunes.

Pat shares his generalist life adventure with his wonderful wife, Christine, who calls him the "Hummus King of Wisconsin," and together they are raising their five children.

More from Pat Flynn

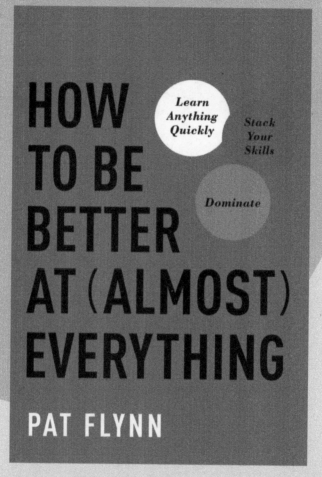

"What Pat presents in this book represents a paradigm shift in the way we all should be approaching our businesses and lives. It's not about killing yourself trying to be the best. It's about putting the puzzle pieces together, getting better at what you need to get better at, and offering something valuable and unique to the marketplace."
—Som Sikdar, CEO of Dragon Gym Martial Arts and Fitness

Available now
where books are sold.